TOP

KETOGENIC

DIET

RECIPES

RWG Publishing

RWG Publishing
PO Box 596
Litchfield, IL 62056
https://rwgpublishing.com/

Published in the United States of America

Table of Contents

SCHNITZEL

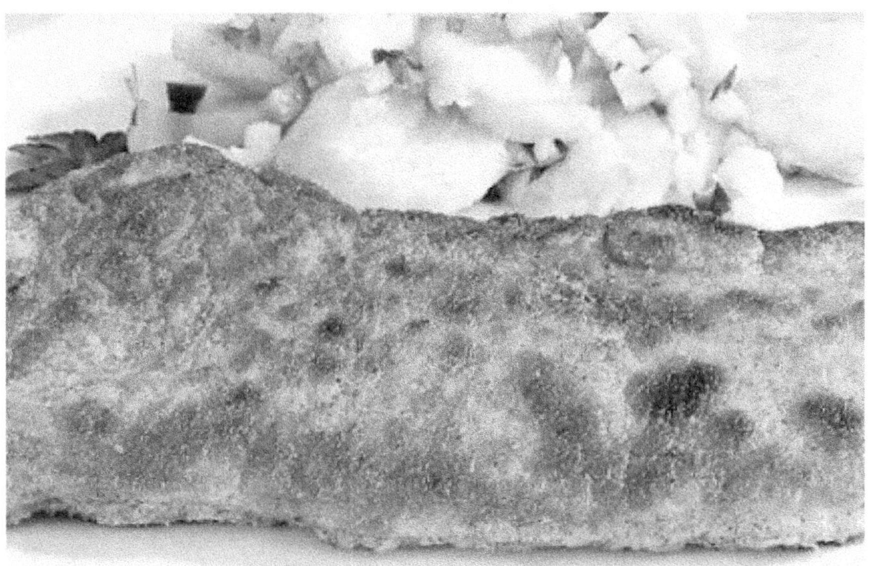

Ingredients for 4 portions

- 600 g   Veal schnitzel (from leg or top shell)
- 3   Egg
- Salt
- 250 g   clarified butter
- Lemon, cut into wedges
- Flour, smooth
- Bread crumbs

Preparation

Total time approx. 50 minutes

1. Have the butcher cut beautiful veal cutlets and cut them lightly at the edges. Cover the schnitzel with cling film and gently plate (tap). The thickness of the schnitzel is individually tailored to your personal taste, but usually measures approx. 6 mm. Salt the cutlets evenly on both sides.
2. Gently whisk the eggs with a fork. Turn the veal cutlets in flour on both sides, pull through the eggs and then turn in breadcrumbs, gently pressing on the breadcrumbs. Gently shake off the schnitzel and remove excess crumbs.
3. Heat plenty of clarified butter in a suitable pan to a height of approx. 2 - 3 cm. Place the cutlets in the hot fat and brown them while repeatedly swinging the pan. Then turn carefully using a meat fork and finish baking from the other side. Lift out of the pan with a baking scoop.
4. Drain the schnitzel, dab off the excess fat with kitchen paper and serve garnished with a lemon wedge.
5. Suitable side dishes are potato salad, cucumber salad, lamb's lettuce or parsley potatoes.

BRAISED BEEF WITH VINEGAR AND CREAM

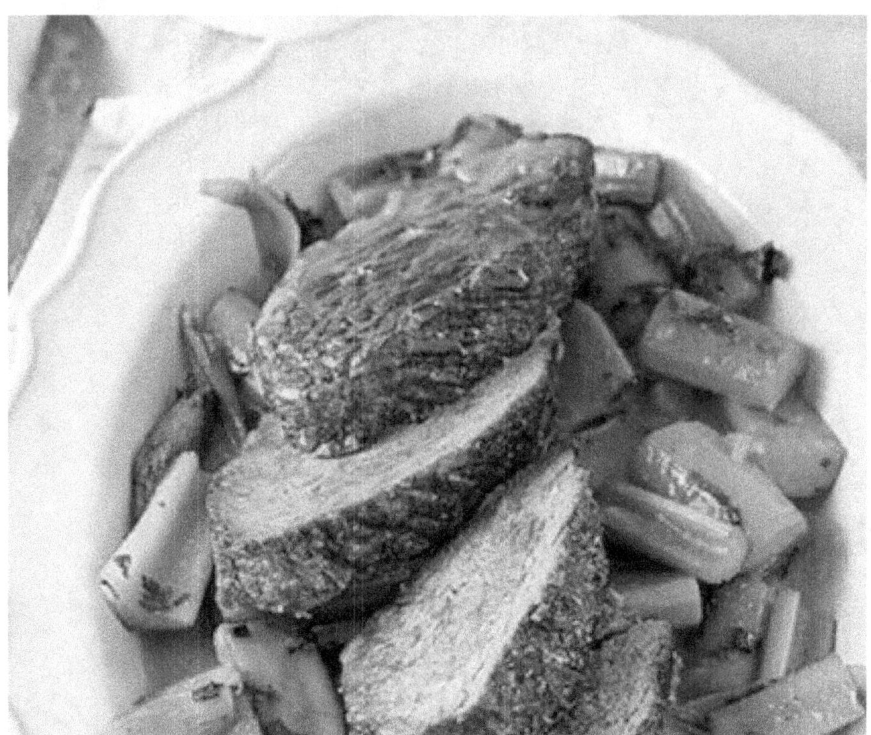

Ingredients for 4 portions

- 3 tbsp. butter
- 800 g   Roast beef (shoulder or other stew)
- 1 tbsp. Flour
- 1 small Onion, quartered
- 50 ml   Wine vinegar or balsamic vinegar
- Salt and pepper
- 200 ml Meat soup
- 100 ml cream

Preparation

Total time approx. 3 hours 30 minutes

1   Heat the butter in a not too big saucepan. Dust the piece of meat with flour, add it with the quartered onion and fry well on all sides. Make sure that the onions do not become too dark. Pour in the vinegar and let it evaporate completely. Sprinkle the meat with salt and freshly ground pepper. Pour in the broth first, then the cream. Put a tight lid on, reduce the heat and braise the meat for about 3 hours.

2   At the end of the cooking time, cut the meat into pieces, arrange and pour the nicely tied sauce on top.

3   The original side dish is mashed potatoes or creamed potatoes with steamed vegetables.

MEATLOAF THE ITALIAN WAY

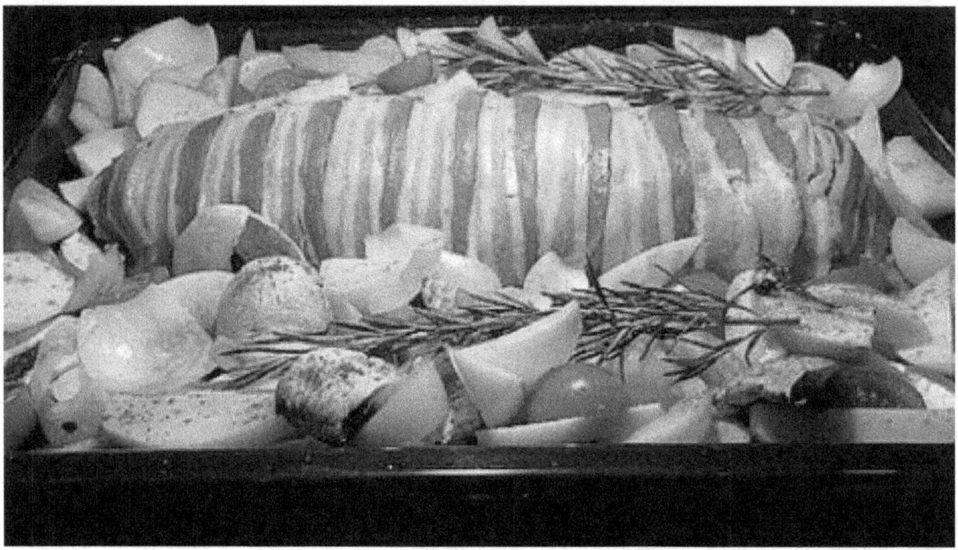

Ingredients for 4 portions

- 500 g   minced meat
- Buns, stale
- Onion
- Egg
- Salt and pepper
- Basil shredded
- For the filling:
- 100 g   Olives, black, without stones
- 100 g   Tomato, dried out of a glass
- Clove of garlic, more at will
- 250 g   Mozzarella
- 100 g   Parma ham, in thin slices

Preparation

Total time approx. 1 hour 10 minutes

1   Put the minced meat in a bowl for the meat dough. Soak the bun well now.
2   Finely chop the onion and add to the minced meat along with the egg. Squeeze out the bread roll and tear it apart, also add to the minced meat. Knead everything into a malleable meat batter and season well. Squeeze out on cling film to a plate of about 30 x 20 cm. The plate should be about 1 cm thick.
3   /Cut the olives and tomatoes into strips for the filling. Chop the cloves of garlic and dice the mozzarella. Mix well and sprinkle on the meat batter. Leave a margin of at least 2 cm if possible. Now carefully roll up the minced meat plate using the film and place it on a baking sheet. It shouldn't tear down. Round off a bit at the ends. Preheat the oven to 180 ° C.
4   In the meantime, place the ham around the roast so that it is completely covered.
5   Then bake the meatloaf for about 30-40 minutes.

6   Use a roaster to lift off the tray onto a plate and serve while still hot.
7   Fresh ciabatta or risotto goes well with this.

FRANCONIAN SHOVEL

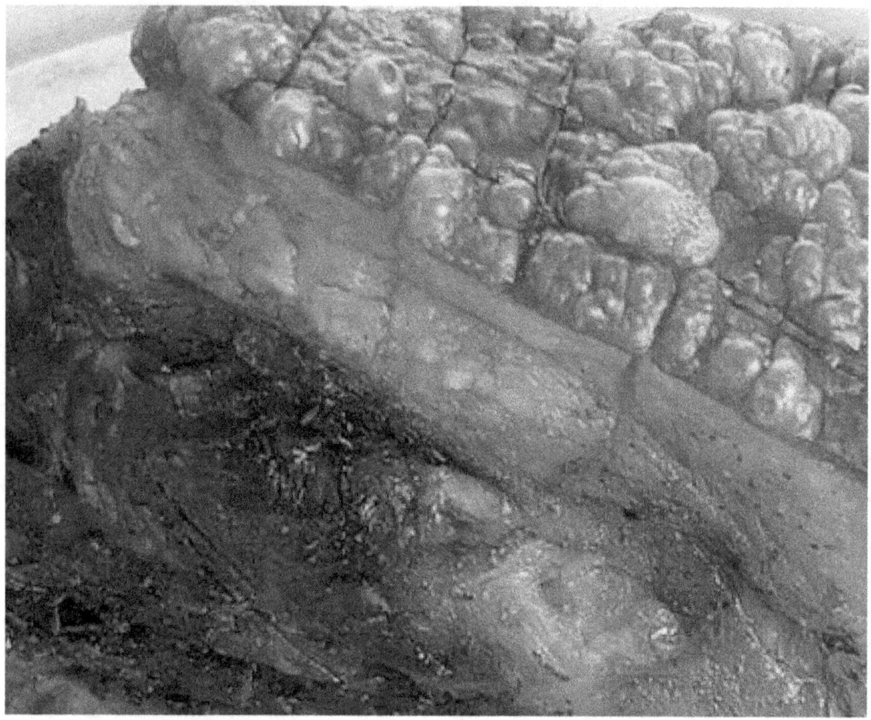

Ingredients for 4 portions

- 1½ kg   Pork (shoulder with bones and rind - shovel)
- Salt and pepper
- 1 teaspoon   Caraway seed
- 1 tbsp. clarified butter
- 1 large Onion
- 1 large Carrot
- Beer, dark

Preparation

Total time approx. 2 hours 30 minutes

1   Cut the rind of the roast pork diagonally or have it cut while shopping.

2   Wash the roast pork, pat dry and rub thoroughly with salt and pepper. Heat the fat in an iron casserole and fry the roast on all sides.

3   Quarter the onion and cut the carrot into large pieces. Pour in 1 cup of water. Push the roast onto the lower rail in the oven preheated to 200 degrees and fry with the rind upwards with occasional watering with the roast juice in 1 1 / 2-2 hours. Possibly. Pour some more water. Brush the last 30 minutes with beer so that the crust becomes nice and crispy.

4   Take out the roast and let it stand for 10 minutes.

5   Deglaze the gravy with a little water, pour through a sieve, degrease and possibly season with a little salt, possibly bind a little. (I bind my sauce by mashing the vegetables first and then passing the sauce through a sieve. This also gives a fine taste) Sufficient for frying.

6   Side dish: potato dumplings and coleslaw.

CRISPY FRIED PORK KNUCKLE

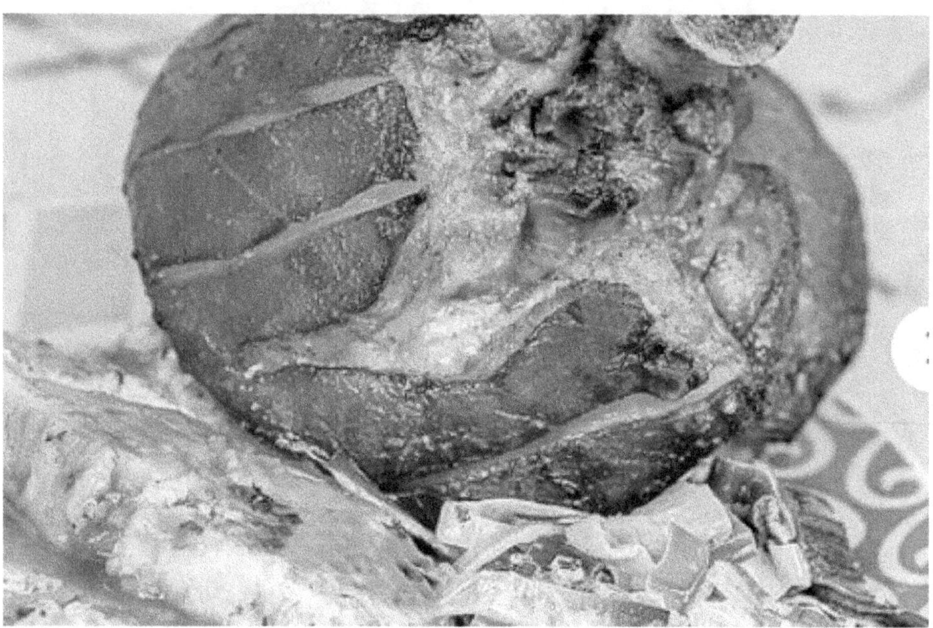

Ingredients for 2 portions

- 1½ kg   Pork
- 2   Onion, peeled and halved
- 5 toes   Garlic, peeled and halved
- Carnation
- bay leaves
- 1 teaspoon   Juniper berry
- ½ tsp   Caraway seed
- 2 Tea spoons   salt
- Pepper, coarser from the mill

Preparation

Total time approx. 2 hours 45 minutes

1   Put water in a large saucepan. Add onions, garlic and the spices. Heat everything, bring to the boil briefly and put the knuckles in the water, they should be covered with water. Approximately let it soak for 90 minutes.

2   Just before the time is up, preheat the oven to 180 to 200 ° C. Remove the knuckles from the water, drain and fry them in the oven for a good hour.

ANTIPASTI MISTI

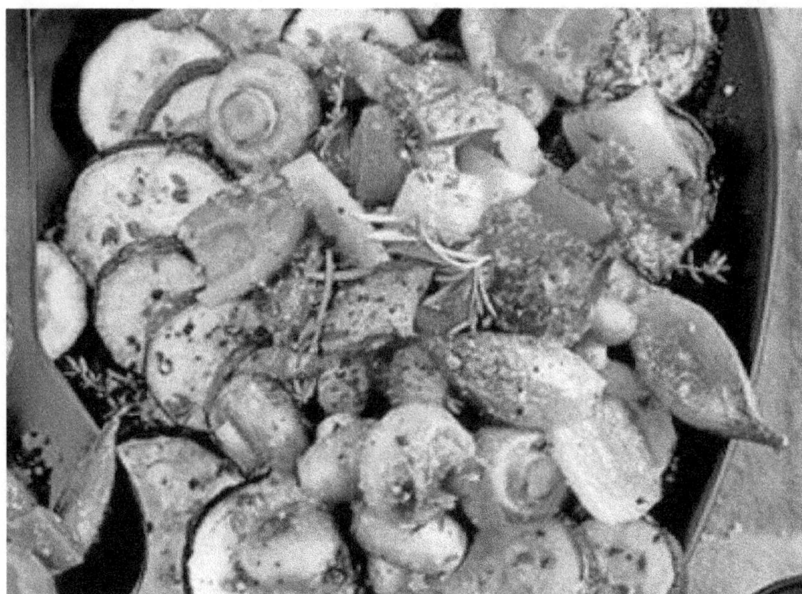

Ingredients for 6 portions

- 1 Eggplant
- 4 m. In size   zucchini
- Bell pepper, yellow, green and red, possibly also pointed pepper
- 500 g   mushrooms
- Shallot
- 250 ml Olive oil, high quality
- 2 tbsp. balsamic
- Rosemary
- Thyme
- Salt
- 1 Chili pepper, fresh, possibly a dried one for the oil
- Garlic cloves

Preparation

Total time approx. 1 hour 25 minutes

1   The marinade should be set at least 24 hours before need. Press the cloves of garlic for this and add them to the olive oil together with the balsamic vinegar. It is best to puree with the help of the magic wand (this way you don't accidentally bite a piece of clove of garlic). Now add a little rosemary and thyme. If you like it a little hotter, you can add a dried chili pepper. If the oil should last longer, keep it in the fridge!

2   Wash the vegetables and cut them into large pieces, "peel" the mushrooms.

3   Preheat the oven to about 180 degrees.

4   Place the vegetables on a deep baking sheet. Salt a little more, pour the chopped chilli, the fresh rosemary and thyme and the prepared oil over it. Approximately Bake for 10 minutes, then switch off the oven, but leave the vegetables in the stove for another 60 minutes.

5   The vegetables go well with a barbecue evening, but also as a starter with an Italian menu or just with a baguette.

HEARTY PEA SOUP

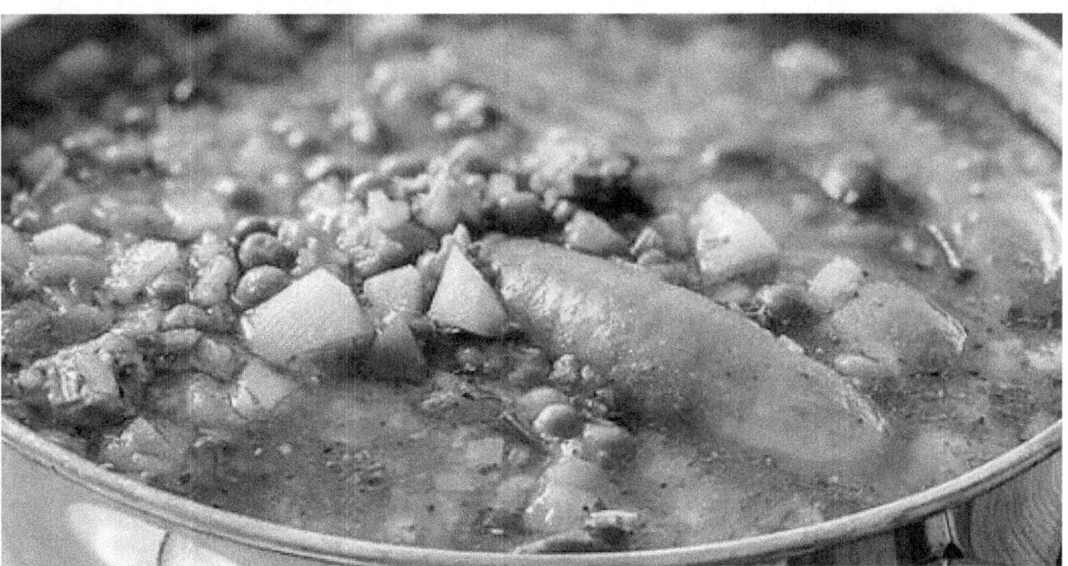

Ingredients for 3 portions

- 150 g Peas, dried
- ½ liter water
- 150 g Bacon, in one piece
- 100 g Leek, cut into thin rings
- 100 g Carrot (roots), finely diced
- 50 g Celery, peeled, in one piece
- 150 g Potato, diced finely
- 1 Bay leaf
- 1 Onion, finely diced
- 1 tbsp. oil
- 250 ml Meat soup
- Pepper
- 250 g Mette ends

Preparation

Total time approx. 14 hours 30 minutes

1. Soak the peas in 1/2 liter of water overnight.
2. Bring to the boil together with the water the next day. After about half an hour, add the bacon and cook everything for another half an hour. Add the leek rings, carrot and potato cubes and the bay leaf. Fry the onion cubes in a small pan in hot oil, then add them to the soup. Add the piece of celery. Add the broth and cook the soup for another half an hour.
3. After this time remove the piece of celery, bay leaf and streaky bacon.

4. Now either puree the soup by hand with a pounder or hold a blender for a short time. Now cut the bacon into small pieces and put it back in the soup, together with the ends of the fat. Season with pepper. Salting is usually not necessary due to the bacon and the fat ends.
5. Finally, let it steep for another half hour on the lowest heat setting, stirring occasionally. Serve hot.

GYROS

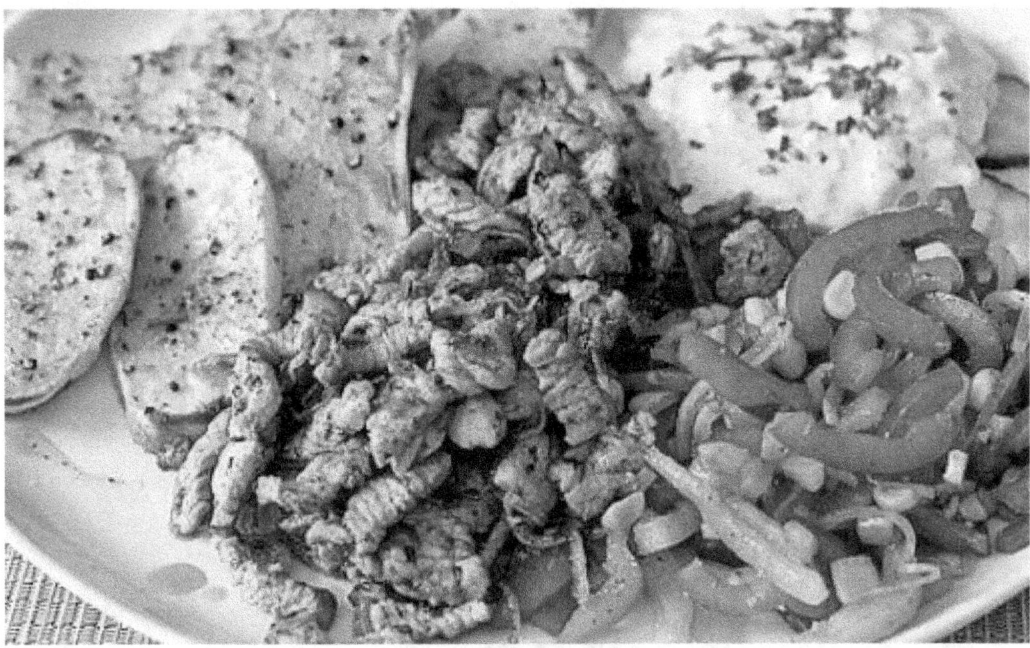

Ingredients for 4 portions

- 600 g   pork cutlet
- 2 Tea spoons   oregano
- 2 Tea spoons   thyme
- 3 tsp   Paprika powder, noble sweet
- 1 teaspoon   Cumin powder
- 2 toes   garlic
- Onion
- salt
- 150 ml olive oil
- 2 splashes   lemon juice
- 1 teaspoon   Mustard, spicy
- Pepper, freshly ground

Preparation

Total time approx. 2 days 40 minutes

1   First wash the meat, pat dry and cut into wafer-thin strips. Peel the onions and cut them into strips. Peel and press the garlic. Mix everything with the spices and marinate in the fridge for about 1 - 2 days.
2   Fry in portions in a very hot pan and keep warm. Serve the gyros hot.
3   Coleslaw, rice and Greek antipasti are enough as side dishes.

DANISH ROAST PORK

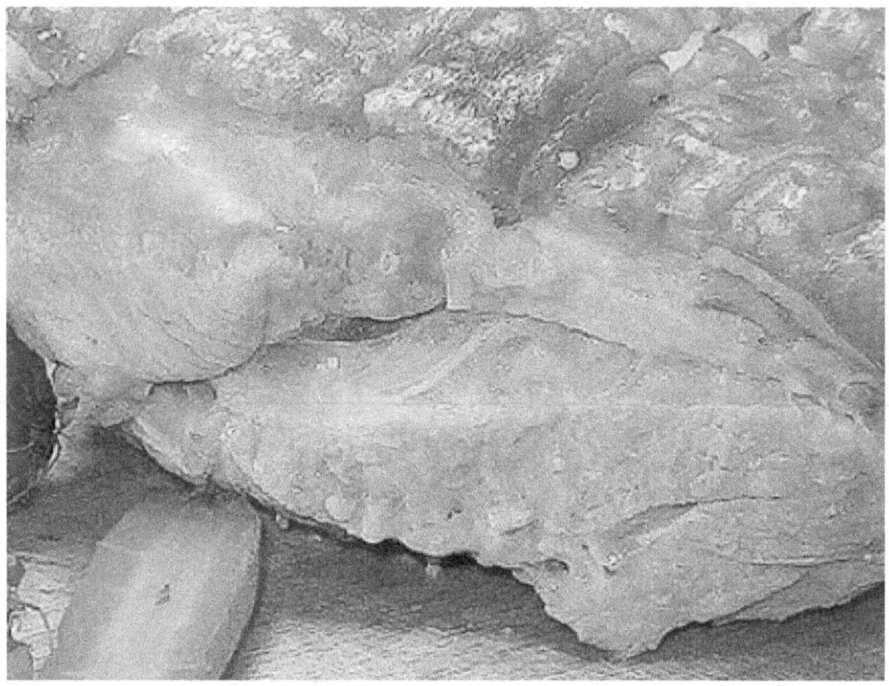

Ingredients for 4 portions

- 1½ kg   Cutlet meat with rind
- 3 bay leaves
- Salt and pepper
- Caraway seed

Total time approx. 4 hours 40 minutes

1   Cut the rind into parallel strips with a sharp knife. Only cut in so far that the fat layer is touched. Fill a plate with approx. 2 cm of water, place the roast in the water with the rind down and leave it there for 2 hours. Only the rind may be in the water.
2   Lightly salt the roast, but rub salt well between the rind strips. Put 3 bay leaves between the rind strips. Pepper the roast lightly, add a little cumin. Put the roast on a rack, add some water to the clean. Fry for one and a half hours at 180 degrees, then another 10 minutes at high temperature. Let the roast rest for 15 minutes without covering the rind so that it stays crispy.
3   Drain the gravy, boil it down, season to taste and if necessary bind with Mondawmin.
4   This goes with glazed Danish potatoes or dumplings.

FILLED MUSHROOMS

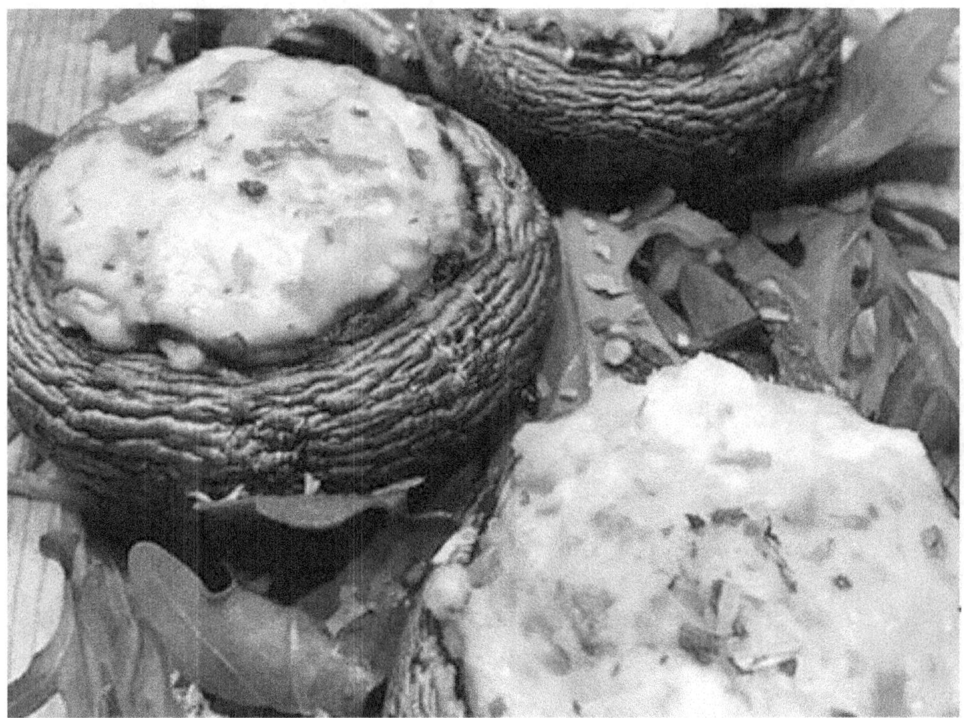

Ingredients for 4 portions

- 500 g Mushrooms, big
- 200 g Ham, (serrano)
- 1 m Onion
- 2 Clove of garlic (at will)
- 200 g Crème fraiche with herbs
- 3 tbsp. sweet cream
- Salt and pepper
- 250 g Cheese, grated (Manchego)
- Oil

Preparation

Total time approx. 30 minutes

1 Clean the mushrooms and remove the stems.
2 Cut the onion, cloves of garlic, Serrano ham and the stems very small. Briefly fry everything together in a pan in a little oil, add crème fraiche and cream. Stir well and season with pepper and salt. Approximately Mix in 100 g of Manchego.
3 Place the mushrooms in a greased baking dish and spread the mass over the cavities. Sprinkle with the remaining cheese and bake at 180 degrees for 20-30 minutes in a preheated oven.

PESTO ROSSO

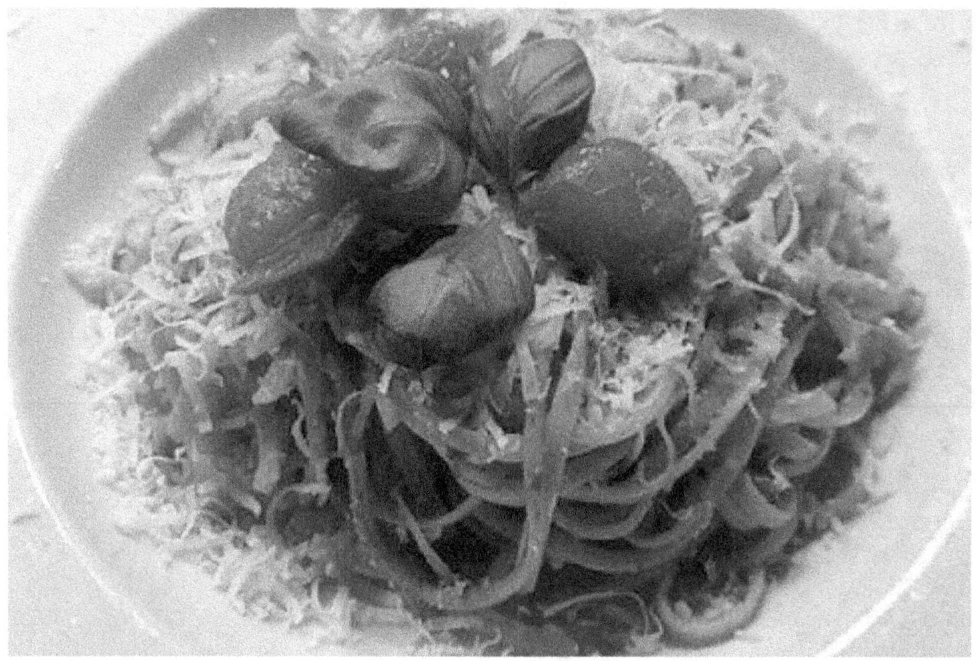

Ingredients for 4 portions

- 150 g   Tomato, sun-ripened dried
- 150 ml Olive oil, fruity mild
- 1 toe   garlic
- 20 sheets   Basil, great fresh
- 50 g   Parmesan, Grana Padano or old Pecorino
- 30 g   Pine nuts or almond sticks
- 1 small Chili pepper, mild red
- 3 tbsp. Red wine, dry, alternatively beetroot juice
- 1 tbsp., heaped tomato paste
- Salt and pepper, black, freshly ground

Preparation

Total time approx. 10 minutes

1   Peel and roughly chop the garlic, wash the basil, dry and chop it roughly, remove the stalk from the stalk, core and chop it roughly, chop the dried tomatoes roughly, chop the cheese as well.
2   Put all ingredients in a blender jar, fill up with oil and mix vigorously with the blender stick. Season with salt and pepper.

POINTED PEPPER - BOAT

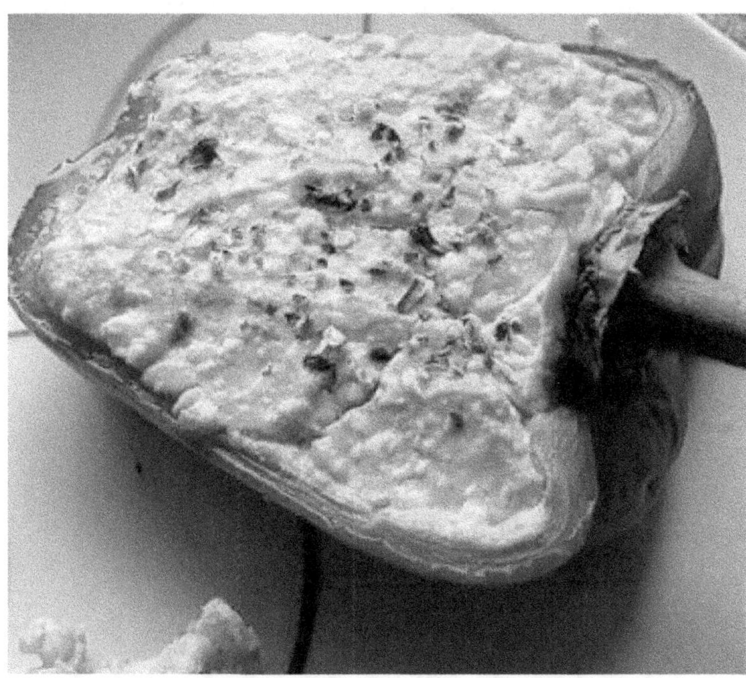

Ingredients for 1 portions

- 500 g Pointed peppers, red
- 200 g feta cheese
- 3 tbsp. Crème fraiche, heaped
- 2 toes Garlic, depending on the size also 3
- 1 tbsp. tomato paste
- Salt
- Pepper
- Olive oil

Preparation

Total time approx. 15 minutes

1. Halve the peppers, remove the stalk and core.
2. For the cream, crumble the sheep's cheese in a bowl and stir well with the remaining ingredients until a smooth mass is formed. Season to taste and fill the pepper halves evenly.
3. Place the filled boats on a sheet of baking paper and drizzle with olive oil.
4. Bake in the oven at 200 ° C for about 20-30 minutes. The peppers start to brown slightly and the scent announces when they are done.
5. The grill option for summer:
6. Remove the stalks from the pointed peppers and remove the stones, but do not halve them. Fill with the cream and wrap tightly in aluminum foil and place on the grill.

CATALAN SEAFOOD POT

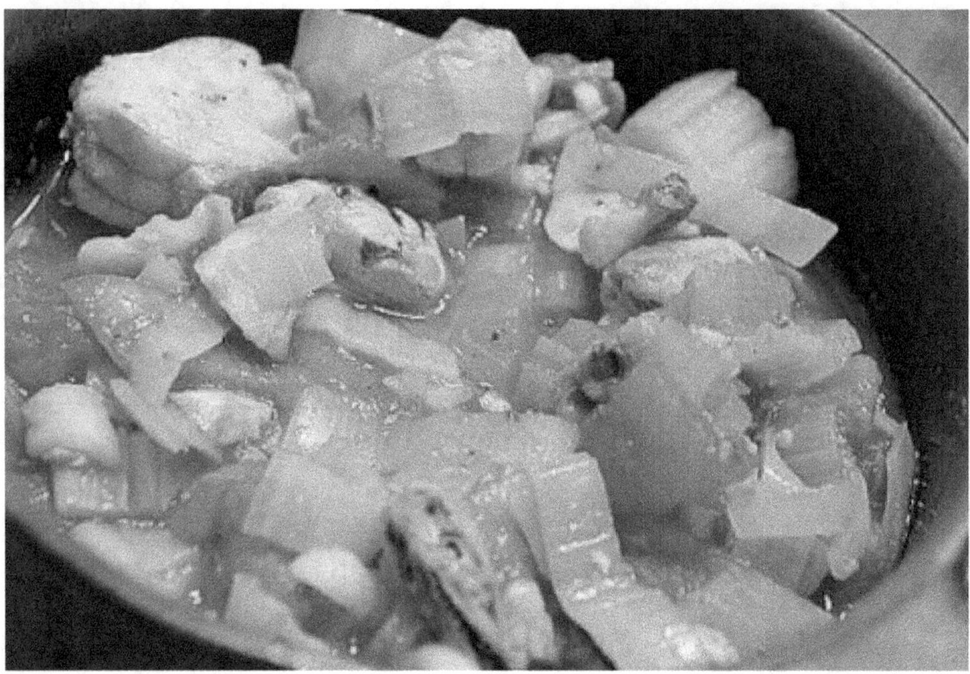

Ingredients for 2 portions

- 1 m   Onion
- 1 bar   leek
- 1 tbsp. olive oil
- 1 toe   garlic
- 1 can   Tomato, peeled (400 g)
- 100 ml White wine, drier, more Spanish
- 250 g   Seafood, mixed, frozen
- 250 g   Fish fillet
- Salt and pepper, black, freshly ground
- 1 small Dose saffron
- 1 teaspoon   Chili flakes, dried
- 2 tbsp. Sherry, drier

Preparation

Total time approx. 40 minutes

1   Allow fish and seafood to thaw slowly.
2   Peel and dice the onion. Clean, cut, wash and cut the leek into rings.
3   Heat the oil in a saucepan, peel the garlic, chop and add. Stir in the onions and the leek and sauté. Chop the tomatoes a little and add with the juice, if necessary, crush them a little.
4   Pour in the white wine and stir in the seafood. Season with salt, pepper, saffron and chili flakes. Cover and simmer for 10 minutes, stirring occasionally.
5   In the meantime, wash the fish fillet cold and dry it, dice it bite-size and season it with salt and pepper.

6   Refine the seafood pot with sherry, stir in the fish cubes, set the cooker to the lowest setting
        and let everything rest for about 7 minutes.
7   Enjoy low carb without any side dishes.

SZEGED GOULASH

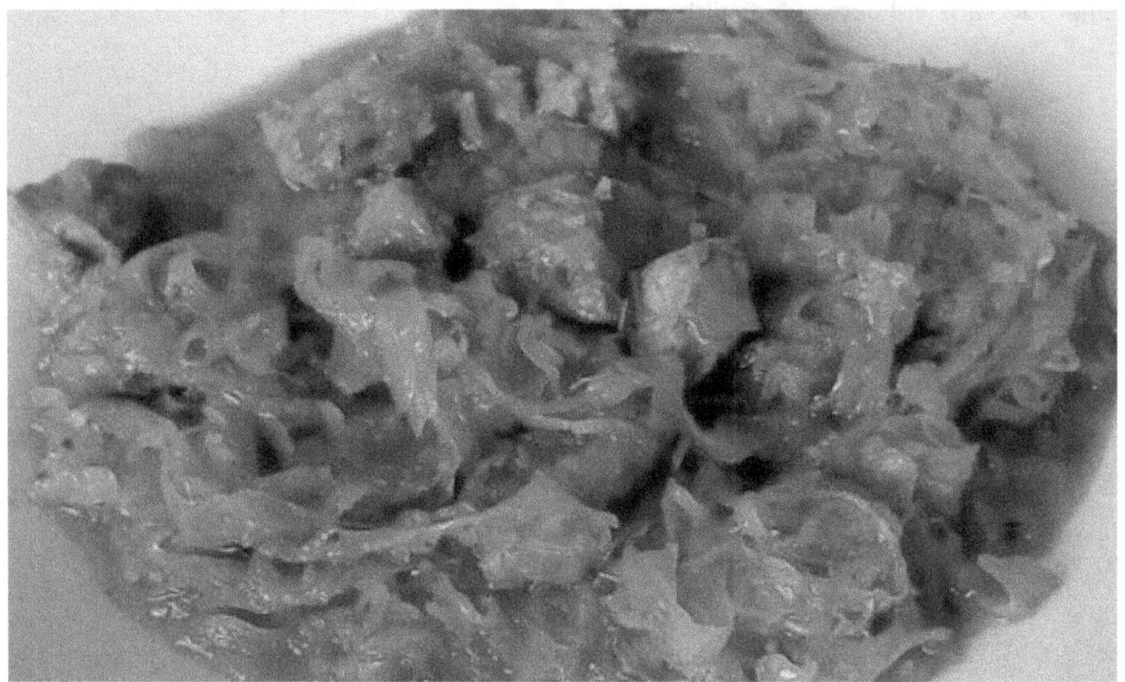

Ingredients for 6 portions

1	250 g	Onion
2	300 g	pork meat
3	300 g	beef
4	100 g	Bacon, streaky
5	500 g	sauerkraut
6	500 ml	Meat soup

- 1 tbsp. tomato paste
- 1 cup   Crème fraiche Cheese
- 2 Tea spoons   food starch
- 1 teaspoon   Paprika powder, spicy
- Salt and pepper
- 2 tbsp. water

Preparation

Total time approx. 30 minutes

1. Peel the onion and cut it into slices. Wash the meat, dry it and cut it into 2 cm cubes.
2. Cut the bacon into cubes and skip it. Add the onion and sauté in it for about 5 minutes. Add the paprika powder and the tomato paste and stir in. Now add the meat and season with salt and pepper. Put the sauerkraut on the meat. Pour broth over everything and let it simmer for about 1.5 hours.
3. Then stir in crème fraiche. Mix the cornstarch with 2 tablespoons of water and bind the goulash with it. Season again with salt and pepper. Serve hot.

ASPARAGUS FROM THE OVEN

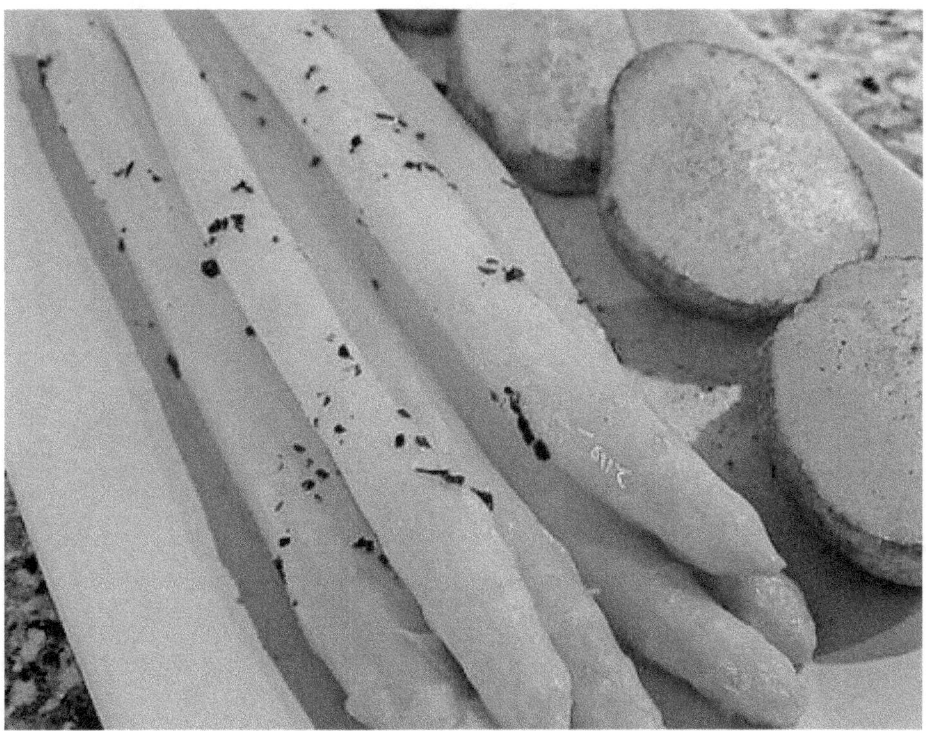

Ingredients for 3 portions

- 1½ kg   Asparagus, white
- 1 pinch sugar
- 1 teaspoon   salt
- ½ tsp   Pepper, freshly ground
- 150 g   butter
- White wine or rosé wine
- ½ half   Lemon, juice from it
- Chives

Preparation

Total time approx. 1 hour 20 minutes

1   The preparation time does not take longer than with cooked asparagus, only the cooking time is longer. However, you will be rewarded for this, because the taste is significantly stronger, since the aroma is not overcooked, but the asparagus cooks in its own juice.
2   Preheat the oven to 200 degrees top / bottom heat (convection 180 degrees).
3   Wash and peel the asparagus and cut off the asparagus ends. Place the asparagus, the thicker stalks first, in a baking dish. Sprinkle sugar, salt and pepper over it and cover the asparagus with thin slices of butter. Drizzle with some wine. Close the baking dish completely with aluminum foil and slide it onto the middle rail in the oven. Cook for 60 minutes, then even the thickest sticks are done. If you like the asparagus with a little more bite, cook only for 30 minutes.

4	Melt the rest of the butter in a saucepan, mix with the asparagus broth from the baking dish, a little lemon juice and chives and pour this sauce over the asparagus when serving.

DANISH MEATBALLS

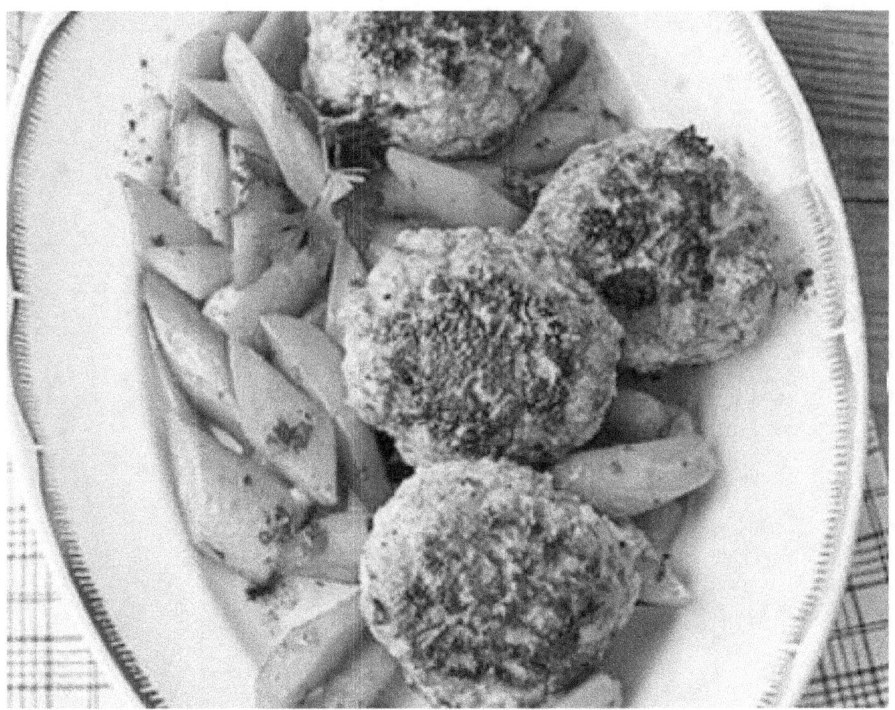

Ingredients for 2 portions

- 300 g   ground pork
- 1 Onion
- 1 Egg
- 1 teaspoon   salt
- Milk, lukewarm
- ½   Bread from the previous day (alternatively bread crumbs)
- 2 Tea spoons   mustard
- 2 tbsp. butter
- 1 teaspoon   pepper

Preparation

Total time approx. 20 minutes

1   Crumble the bun in a bowl and add lukewarm milk so that a soft mass is created. Then add and mix as follows: 1 egg, a short teaspoon of salt and pepper, 1-2 teaspoons of mustard, 1 finely chopped onion and the minced meat. Mix everything well so that a relatively solid mass is formed.

2   Do not let it stand, but immediately heat butter in a pan and form the meatballs from the mixture. Put in the hot fat and fry until they are brown on all sides. Afterwards, do not pour the roast broth away, but add it to the side dish (in Denmark these are mostly jacket potatoes).

3   This goes very well with cooked carrots or spinach.

SPANISH SKEWERS

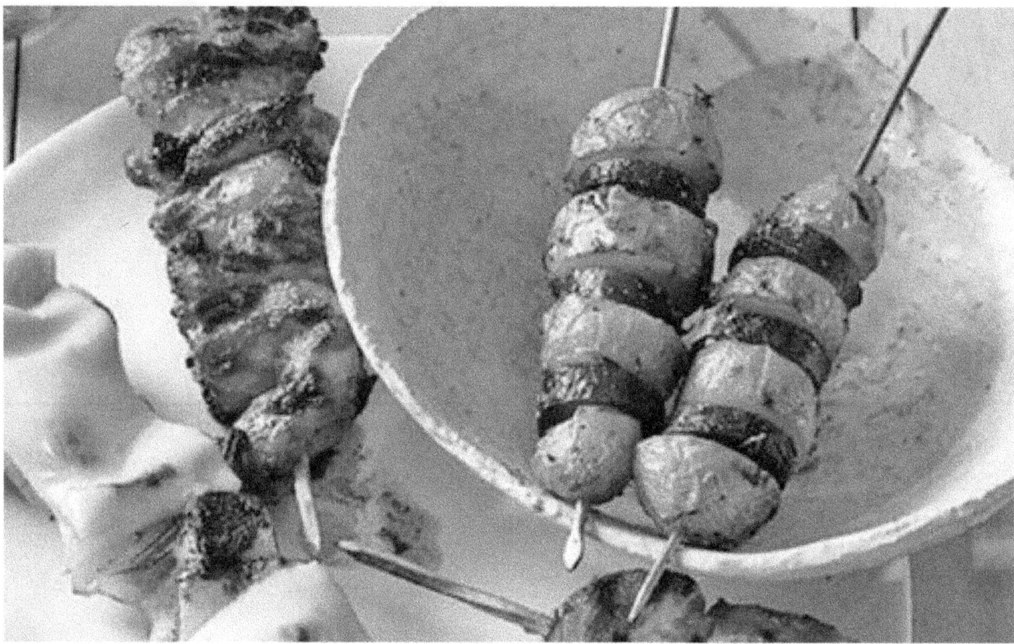

Ingredients for 2 portions

- 250 ml Olive oil or sunflower oil
- Garlic cloves
- 1 small Onion
- Bell pepper, red
- ½ tsp   pepper
- 1 teaspoon   salt
- 4 tsp   chili powder
- 2 Tea spoons   paprika
- 3 tbsp. sugar
- 4 Chicken breast fillet
- oil

Preparation

Total time approx. 2 hours 30 minutes

Cut the onion, garlic and bell pepper into small pieces. Place in a mixing bowl with the remaining ingredients apart from the meat and mix well with a hand blender.

Cut the chicken breast fillets into thin strips and spread them on the wooden skewers. Tip: Dip the skewers in oil before opening.

Finally, put the skewers in the marinade and let them steep for 2-3 hours. The skewers from the grill taste best.

MARINATED ANCHOVIES

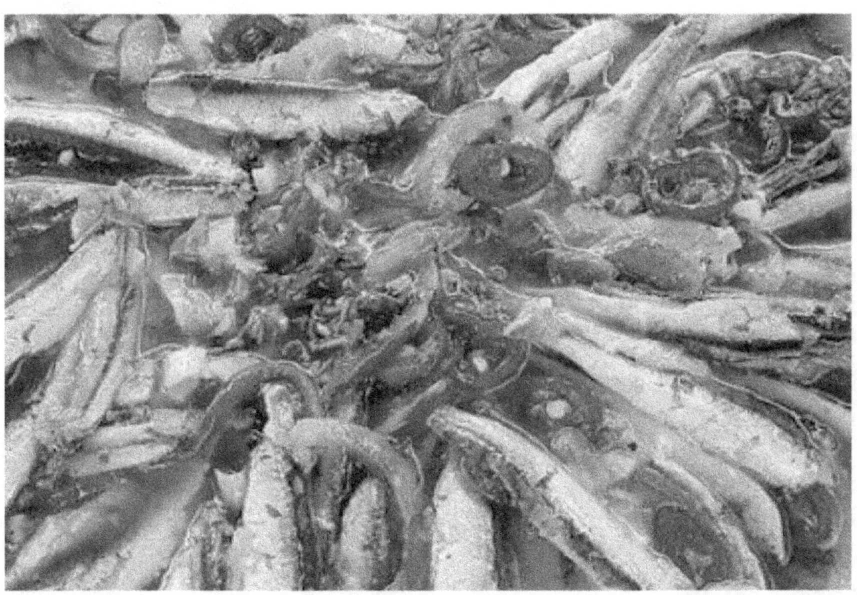

Ingredients for 4 portions

- 500 g   Anchovy fillet, fresh
- 250 ml Vinegar (wine or herbal vinegar), white
- 1 teaspoon   salt
- 4 toes   Garlic, chopped
- 2 tbsp. Parsley, finely chopped

Preparation

Total time approx. 12 hours 30 minutes

1   The head, innards and bones are removed. (After the head is removed, pull the backbone against the tail. This creates two fillets!). Wash and spread in a glass bowl. Cover with vinegar and add salt. Marinate between 8 and 24 hours until the fillets are white and snappy. Then drain the marinade and pour over olive oil and garlic. Sprinkle with parsley.

HAM AND MOZZARELLA PLATE

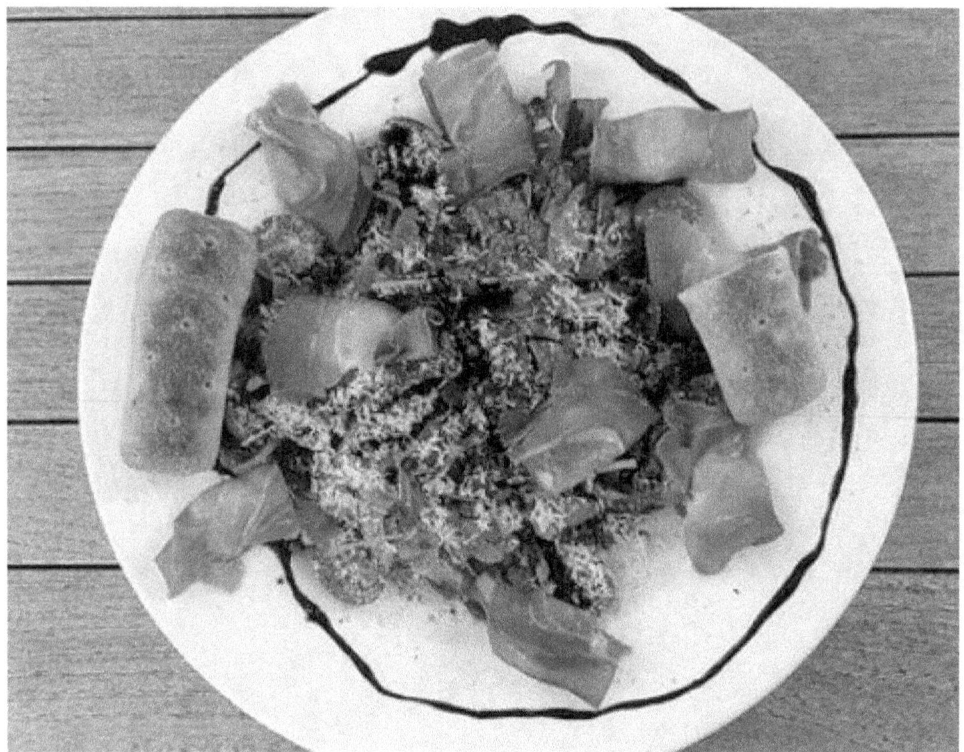

Ingredients for 1 portions

- 125 g   Mozzarella
- 100 g   raw ham, e.g. Parma
- 50 g   arugula
- 4 tsp   olive oil
- 5 cherry tomatoes
- Parmesan cheese, freshly grated
- Balsamic cream, or vinegar
- Salt and pepper

Preparation

Total time approx. 19 minutes

2   Drain the mozzarella and cut lengthwise into four to five slices, each wrapped tightly with a slice of ham.

3   Clean the arugula and tomatoes, then cut the tomatoes into quarters and arrange both ingredients on a plate. Pour the olive oil over the salad and season with salt and pepper.

4   Warm the ham and mozzarella wraps in the oven preheated to 150 ° for about 4 minutes. The mozzarella should soften, but not melt.

5   Now distribute the wraps on the plate and decorate with the balsamic cream and parmesan as you like.

6   Of course, Italian white bread (Ciabatta) also tastes great.

TUSCAN ROAST PORK

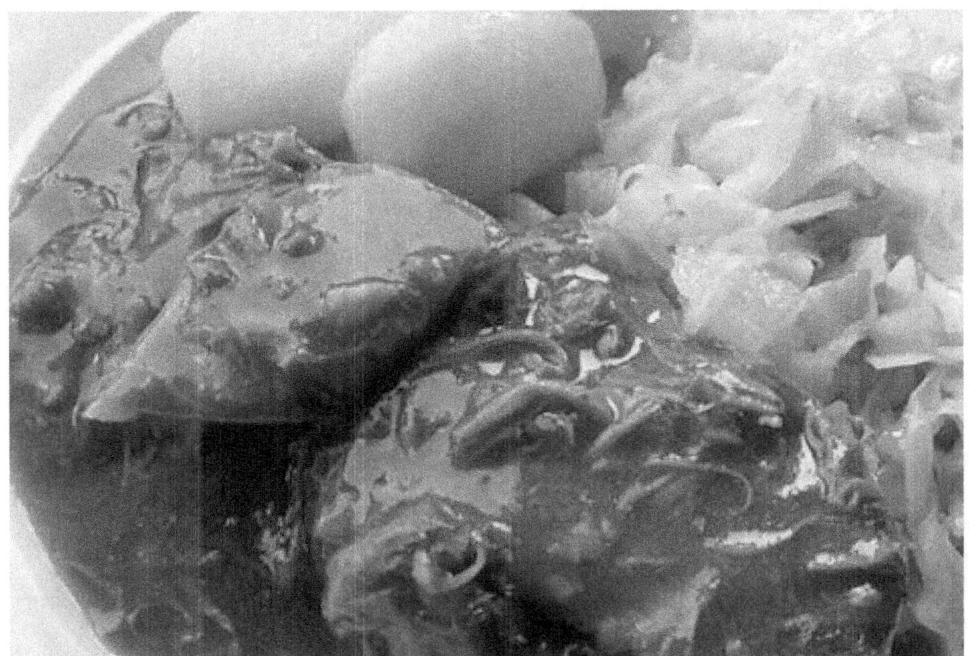

Ingredients for 4 portions

1 kg   pork neck

- 2 Onion
- 2 Garlic cloves
- 10   sage leaves
- 2 Rosemary
- Olive oil
- Butter
- Salt and pepper
- Nutmeg, grated
- 150 ml White wine, drier

Preparation

Total time approx. 2 hours 40 minutes

1   Season the meat vigorously with salt, pepper and grated nutmeg. Then sear well in an olive oil and butter mixture all around.
2   Lift the meat out of the pot and add the chopped onions, garlic and the chopped herbs (sage and rosemary) and also roast vigorously. Add white wine, put the meat back in the pot and reduce the heat to a very low level. Allow the roast to braise for two to three hours, if necessary pour in some wine or broth.
3   Finally cut up the roast and serve with the sauce (I do not pass the sauce through a sieve and do not add any cream either, it is absolutely not necessary). Baked fennel goes well with this.

ALSATIAN SCHNITZEL

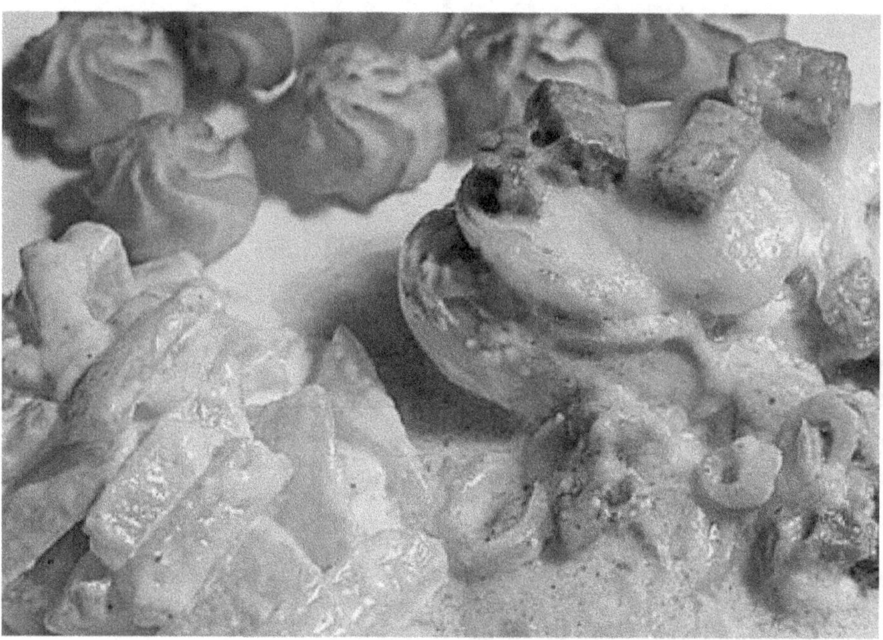

Ingredients for 4 portions

- 600 g   Pork loin or pork fillet, sliced (turkey or chicken is also possible)
- 120 g   Sour cream or crème fraiche
- 120 g   Ham, raw, in cubes
- 1 m   Onion
- 40 g   Cheese, grated (possibly reduced in fat)
- 2 Tea spoons   oil
- Salt and pepper
- Nutmeg

Preparation

Total time approx. 30 minutes

1.   Season the schnitzel and fry briefly in the oil.
2.   Preheat the oven to 200 ° C.
3.   Put the meat in a refractory form and brush with the sour cream (if you like it creamier, you can also use crème fraiche). Cut the onion into rings and spread it with the ham cubes on the chips. Finally sprinkle with a little cheese. Place in the hot oven for about 10 minutes until the cheese has melted.
4.   This goes with baked potatoes (if the oven is on anyway) or noodles with cream sauce.

BEEF FILLET WITH POLENTA STARS AND BACON-WRAPPED BEANS

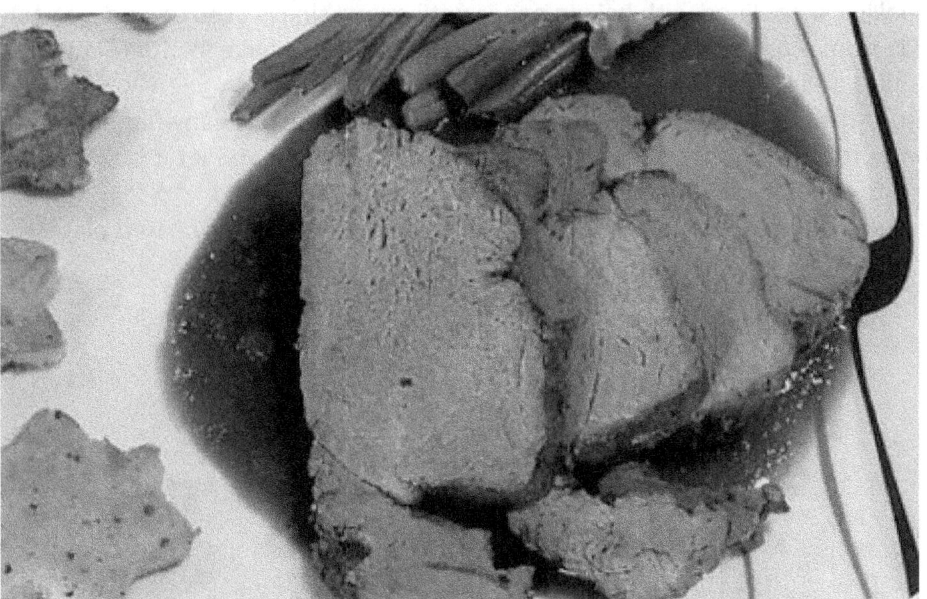

Ingredients for 6 portions

- 1½ kg   Beef
- 500 g   Beans, as long as possible, green (fresh)
- 12 disc Bacon, streaky, thinly sliced
- 180 g   polenta
- 500 ml   vegetable stock
- 3 tbsp. butter
- 4 tbsp. Parmesan cheese, grated
- Thyme and rosemary, some sprigs
- salt and pepper
- Oil for frying
- Onion
- Tomatoes
- 100 ml   red wine
- Gravy

Preparation

Total time approx. 50 minutes

1. Salt and pepper the fillet well, cut the onions and tomatoes into eight and fry everything together with a few sprigs of rosemary and thyme on all sides. Deglaze with approx. 60 ml of red wine. Then continue cooking in a preheated oven at 150 ° C for 30-40 minutes.
2. Bring the vegetable broth to the boil with 1 tablespoon of butter, stir in the polenta and slowly reduce to a firm mass, stirring constantly. Stir in the parmesan, season with salt and pepper, pour onto a baking sheet lined with baking paper and smooth out. Let cool, then cut out stars and fry in the remaining butter on both sides until golden yellow.

3   Put the beans in boiling salted water and cook for 5-8 minutes, so that they are still firm and
        crunchy. Quench immediately in ice water. Then always wrap a few beans with the bacon and
        place them on a baking sheet lined with baking paper until everything is used up and 12 bean
        packages are made from them. Add these to the meat in the oven and bake for 10-15 minutes
        until the bacon is nice and crispy.

4   Take the fillet out of the oven, wrap it in aluminum foil and let it rest. Meanwhile, pass the
        roasting stock, bring to the boil, deglaze with the rest of the red wine and let it boil down a
        little. Season to taste and if necessary add a little sauce binder.

5   Cut the fillet into slices and serve together with the other ingredients on preheated plates.

SPINACH LASAGNA

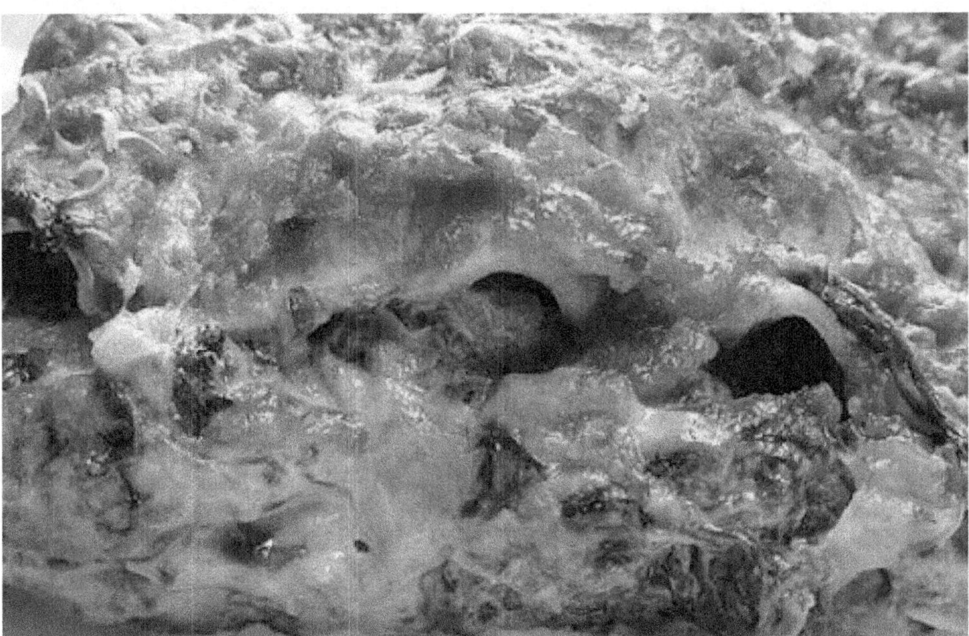

Ingredients for 4 portions

- 800 g   Spinach, frozen or freshly blanched
- 2 m. In size   Onion
- Garlic cloves
- 400 g   Tomato happened
- 2 tbsp. tomato paste
- 2 tbsp. Herbs, mixed, frozen
- Oil
- 350 g   Cream cheese, light
- 100 g   Parmesan
- Salt and pepper
- Nutmeg
- Paprika
- Lasagna plate, as required

Preparation

Total time approx. 1 hour 5 minutes

1   Finely dice the onion and garlic, heat 2 tablespoons of oil and fry half of the onions and garlic in each. Stir in the spinach and let it heat up, then stir in the cream cheese. Season with nutmeg, salt and pepper.

2   Heat 2 tablespoons of oil, fry the remaining onions and the remaining garlic in it, add the tomato paste and herbs, briefly roast and pour the tomatoes on top. Approximately simmer for 5 minutes and season with salt, pepper and paprika powder.

3   Grease a baking dish, spread some tomato sauce in it, then pour the lasagna plates, spinach, tomato sauce and again lasagna plates layer by layer into the mold, finish with tomato sauce. Sprinkle with Parmesan and bake in the preheated oven at 175 ° C for 40 - 45 minutes.

ROSEMARY-BALSAMIC PORK

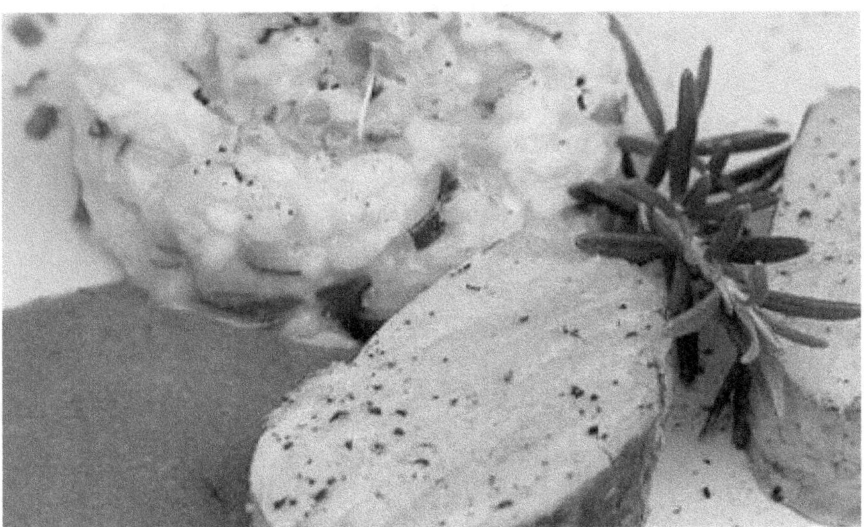

Ingredients for 6 portions

- 1 kg   Pork
- Salt and pepper
- 8 tbsp. White wine, dry
- 4 tbsp. Balsamic, darker
- 4 tbsp. olive oil
- 1 branch   Rosemary, approx. 20 cm, more to taste

Preparation

Total time approx. 20 minutes

1   Salt and pepper the meat. Mix 4 tablespoons of wine and 4 tablespoons of balsamic vinegar. Fry the fillet in oil and continue cooking gently for 10 minutes. Sprinkle with rosemary needles and gradually pour in the wine / vinegar mixture. Let it boil down only a little and always again. After 10 minutes, wrap the fillet tightly in aluminum foil and let it rest.

2   Boil the residue in the pan with the rest of the wine. Cut the meanwhile cooled fillet into thin slices and stir the meat juice remaining in the aluminum foil into the sauce. Drizzle the slices of fillet with the sauce.

3   The amount of sauce can also be increased, the proportion of wine and balsamic vinegar should always remain the same.

4   The fillet is also very warm (i.e. after a short aluminum rest period), but it is absolutely delicious if you pull it through. I take a lot of rosemary because it is really my favorite herb. Newcomers to rosemary should first work with the specified amount.

FETA CREAM WITH PEPPERS AND HERBS

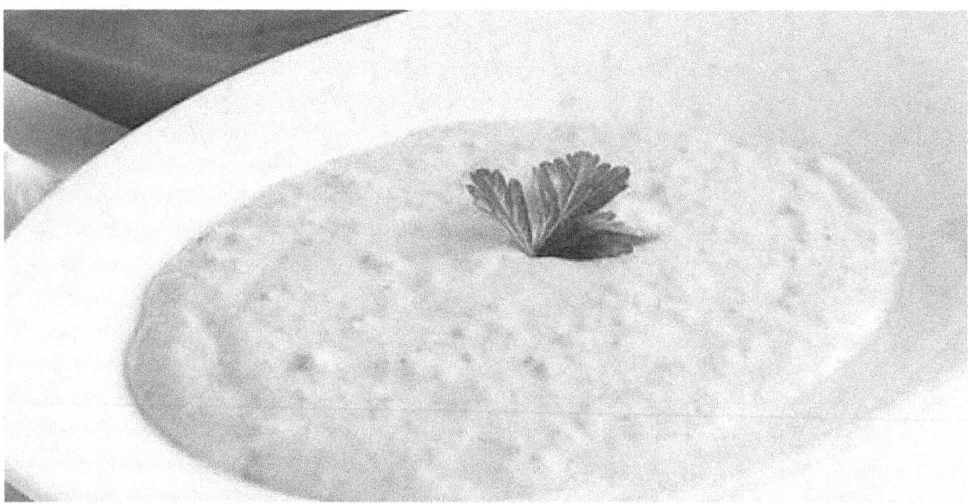

Ingredients for 6 portions

- 200 g   Feta cheese, creamier from cow's milk
- 200 g   Cream cheese, (e.g. Philadelphia)
- Bell pepper, red, small cubes
- 1 teaspoon   herbs of Provence
- ½ tsp   oregano
- 1 tbsp. olive oil
- 3 toes   Garlic, (depending on taste)
- Salt and pepper

Preparation

Total time approx. 4 hours 15 minutes

1   Finely dice the bell pepper and feta cheese. Mix together with the cream cheese and the olive oil with the hand blender to a creamy mass. Add the pressed cloves of garlic and herbs and season with salt and pepper. Refrigerate!

ZURICH SLICED

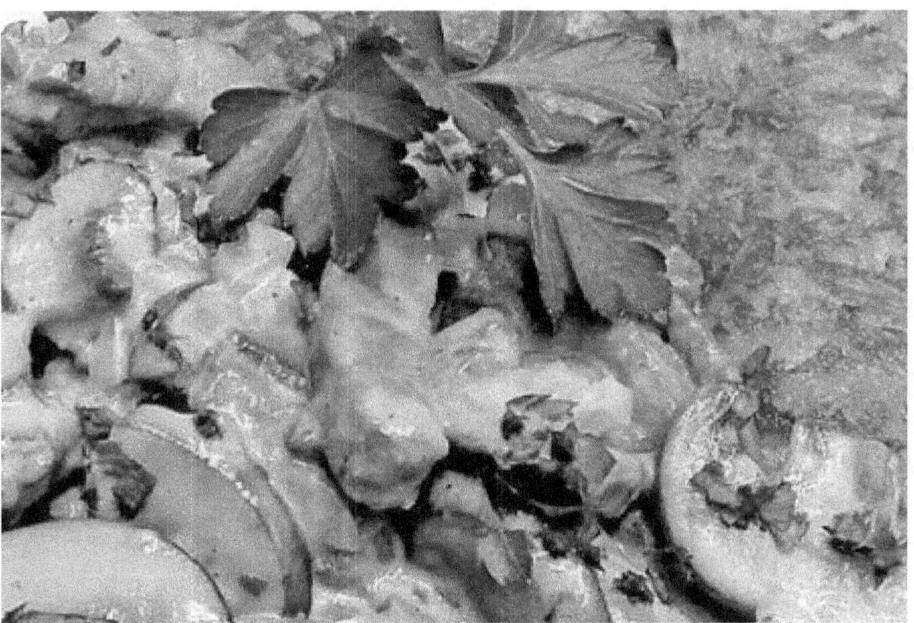

Ingredients for 4 portions

- 4 tbsp. Onion, peeled and chopped
- 160 g   mushrooms
- 560 g   Veal cutlet, hand-sliced (3mm thick)
- Salt
- Pepper, white from the mill
- 1 tbsp. Flour
- 2 tbsp. Oil (peanut oil)
- 3 tbsp. butter
- 200 ml Wine, white
- 400 ml cream

Preparation

Total time approx. 30 minutes

2	Season the sliced meat with salt and pepper from the grinder and divide it into two parts.
3	Heat a large Teflon pan with half of the peanut oil very well, add part of the meat and sauté briefly (!). (Not too long, otherwise the meat will become tough and dry)
4	Take the meat out of the pan, keep warm. Do the same with the rest of the meat.
5	Heat the butter in the same pan, add the onions and stew. Add the sliced mushrooms, dust with the flour and mix. Add white wine and reduce by half. Add the meat juices and the cream and boil everything to the desired consistency. Season with salt and pepper.
6	Put the meat in the sauce (do not cook anymore) and mix.
7	Serve with hash browns.

SOUR TIPS

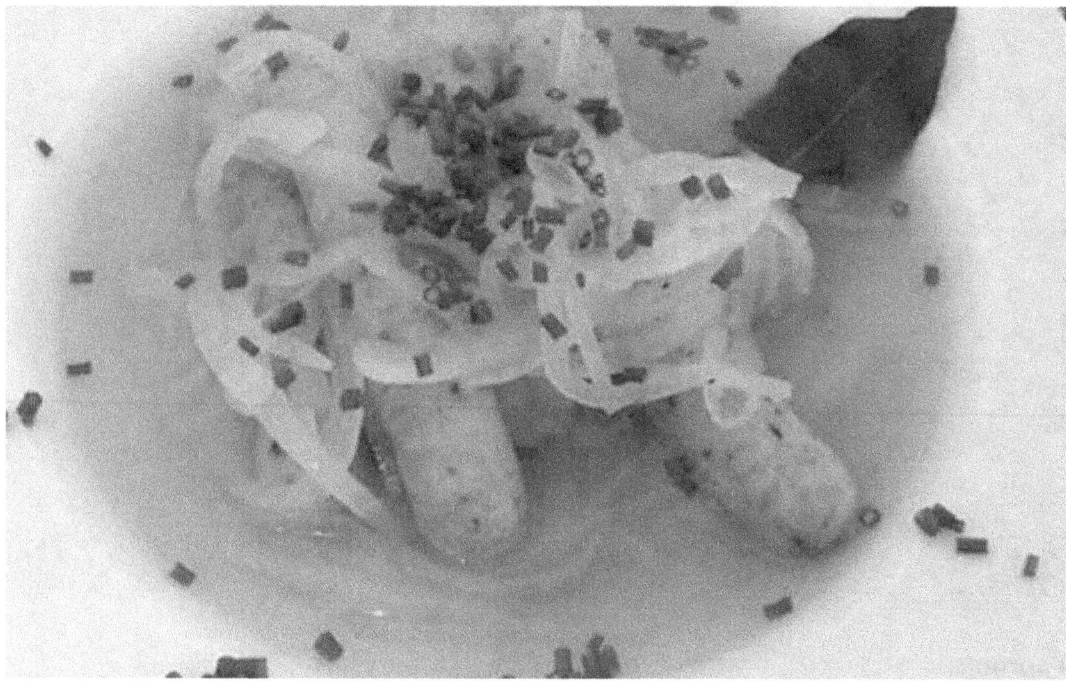

Ingredients for 4 portions

- 24 small ones   Nuremberg grilled sausages, approx. 25 g each
- 1 liter   Meat soup
- 100 ml Vinegar, white (5% acid)
- 6 Juniper berry
- 3 bay leaves
- 30 g   sugar
- 1 teaspoon   Pepper, black from the mill
- 200 ml White wine,
- 4 m. In size   Onion

Preparation

Total time approx. 35 minutes

1   Bring the broth to the boil, add the vinegar, wine and all the spices. Halve the onions, cut into thin slices, add and let simmer for about 15 minutes. Now add the Nuremberg sausages and let them steep for 10 minutes in the low-boiling broth.

2   Put 6 sausages per serving in deep plates or small terrines and scoop some of the broth with onions over it.

3   It goes well with freshly grated horseradish and fresh farm bread.

SCHNINS MINI MEATBALLS

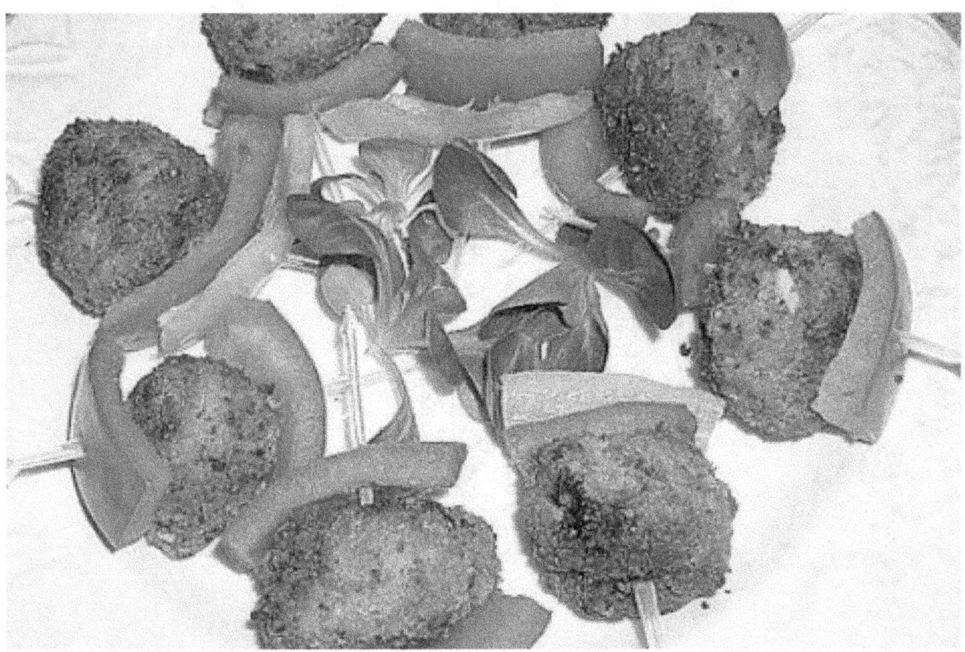

Ingredients for 1 portions

- 500 g   Minced meat, mixed
- 2 Egg S
- 1 Onion, diced finely
- 3 tbsp. bread crumbs
- 2 Clove of garlic, pressed
- Paprika powder, noble sweet
- Mustard
- Salt and pepper

Preparation

Total time approx. 1 hour 25 minutes

1. Mix the minced meat with onions, eggs, breadcrumbs, garlic and mustard thoroughly, season with spicy pepper, mustard, salt and pepper.
2. Shape small balls with wet hands and flatten them a little. Leave in the refrigerator for 1 hour.
3. Fry the meatballs crispy brown on both sides in a pan with hot oil over medium heat.
4. Enjoy warm and cold.

PORK FILLET IN CREAM SAUCE

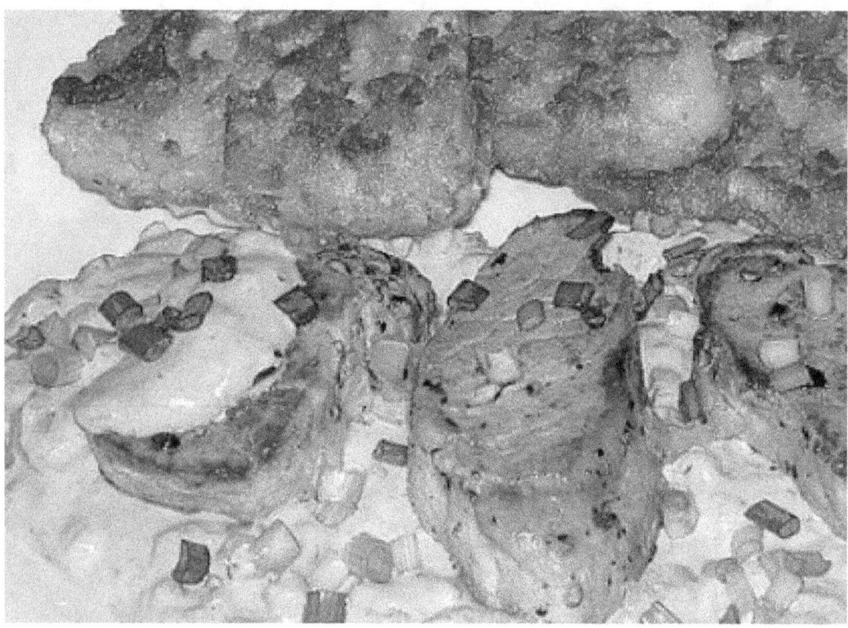

Ingredients for 4 portions

- 150 g   Spring onions
- 800 g   Pork
- 2 tbsp. oil
- 200 g   cream
- 150 ml vegetable stock
- 50 g   Crème fraiche Cheese
- 1 teaspoon   Mustard (Dijon mustard)
- Salt
- Pepper, white

Preparation

Total time approx. 30 minutes

Cut the spring onions into fine rings. Cut the meat into slices about 2-3 cm thick. Heat the oil in the pan. Fry the pork medallions on both sides over high heat, season with salt and pepper and remove. Add the spring onions and sauté briefly. Add the cream, broth, crème fraiche and mustard and bring to the boil. Simmer the meat in the sauce for 5 minutes. Season with salt and pepper.

ROAST BEEF

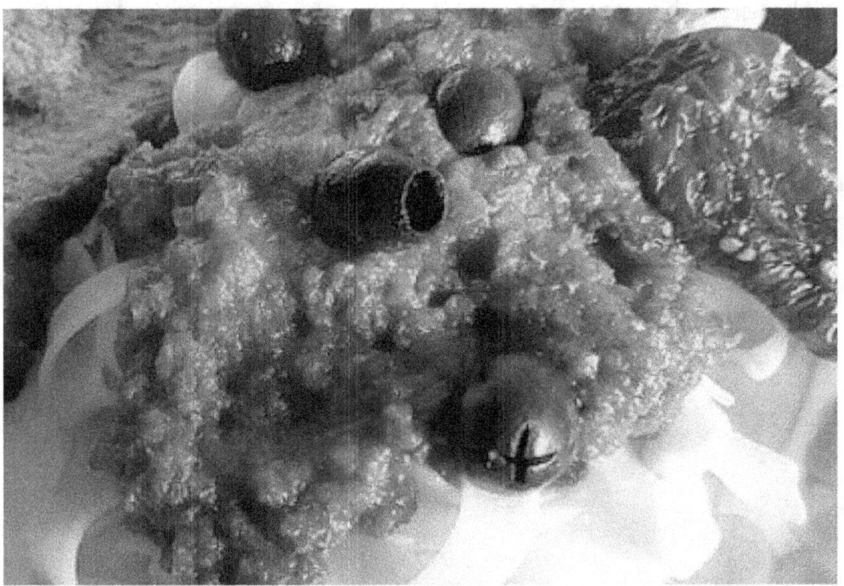

Ingredients for 4 portions

- 1.4 kg   Beef, (from shoulder or leg)
- 2 small ones   Carrot
- 3 bars   celery
- Onion
- 100 g   Bacon, streaky
- 10   Tomato, dried, finely diced
- 10   Olives, dry pickled black, pitted and finely diced
- 300 ml Wine, red, dry (e.g. Sangiovese)
- 500 ml Vegetable broth or poultry broth
- 2 branch   rosemary
- 2 branch   thyme
- 1 Bay leaf
- 2 Clove of garlic, peeled
- ½ tsp   Pepper, whole, roughly pounded in a mortar
- 5 Allspice, whole, roughly pounded in a mortar
- Salt and pepper

Preparation

Total time approx. 45 minutes

1   Preheat the oven to approx. 180 degrees.
2   Finely dice the carrots, celery, onions and bacon.
3   Season the meat with a little salt and pepper and sear well in a roaster with a little oil all
         around. Take out and roast the vegetables in it.
4   Add the bacon, tomatoes and olives and fry briefly. Add the meat again and deglaze with a
         dash of red wine. When the red wine is reduced like a syrup, pour a little more. Repeat until

the red wine is used up. Then pour in the broth and add the spices. Salt if at all, since the bacon and the dried tomatoes are already salty.

5   Close the roaster and let it braise in the oven for at least 3 hours at 180 degrees until the roast is nice and tender.

6   Take out the meat and keep it warm. Fish the rosemary and thyme sprigs and the bay leaf out of the sauce. Reduce the sauce a little more and season with a little salt if necessary. If you like the sauce, you can either bind it with cornstarch or puree some of the vegetables.

7   Cut the meat into slices and serve with the sauce and wide ribbon pasta.

GYROS SOUP

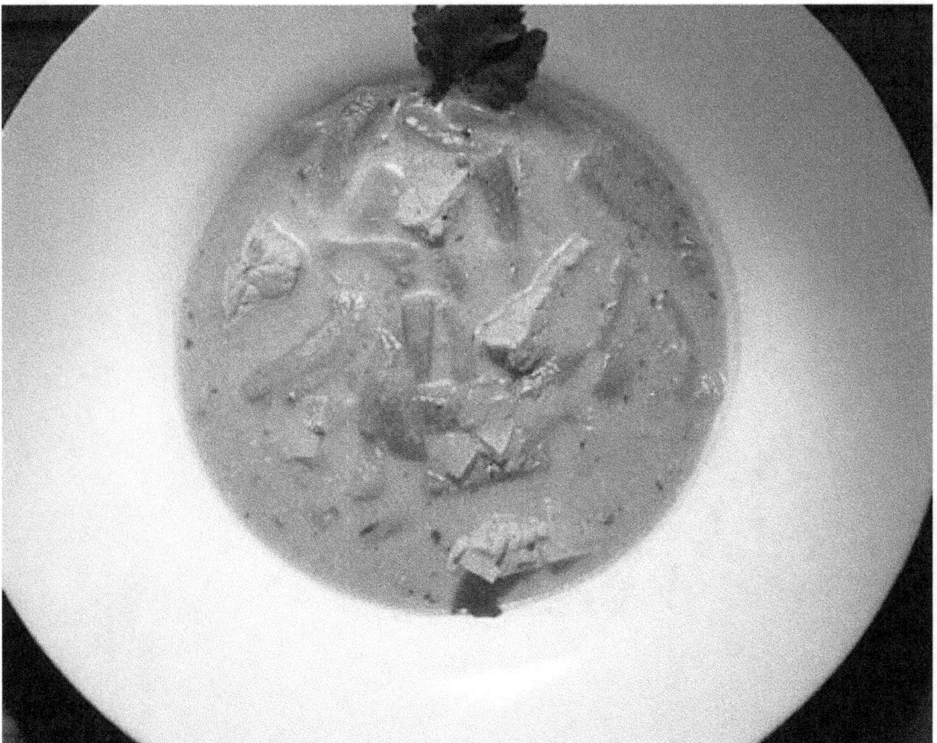

Ingredients for 12 portions

- 1,500 g Meat (gyros)
- 600 ml cream
- 4 Onion, diced
- 3 Bell pepper, green, cut into strips
- 3 Bell pepper, red, cut into strips
- 1 liter   broth
- 500 ml Sauce (gypsy or chili sauce)
- 175 g   cheese spread
- 4 tbsp. olive oil
- Salt and pepper
- Garlic
- Paprika
- Curry powder

Preparation

1   Total time approx. 30 minutes
2   Fry the meat in a large saucepan with the heated olive oil. Add the diced onions and the peppers cut into strips. Let it simmer. Pour in the water. Add the cream, gypsy sauce or chili sauce and processed cheese. Season with the spices as needed. Let it cook until the meat is cooked.
3   Can be prepared well in advance. Just warm up for the party.

MARINATED GOAT CHEESE WITH TARRAGON AND PARSLEY

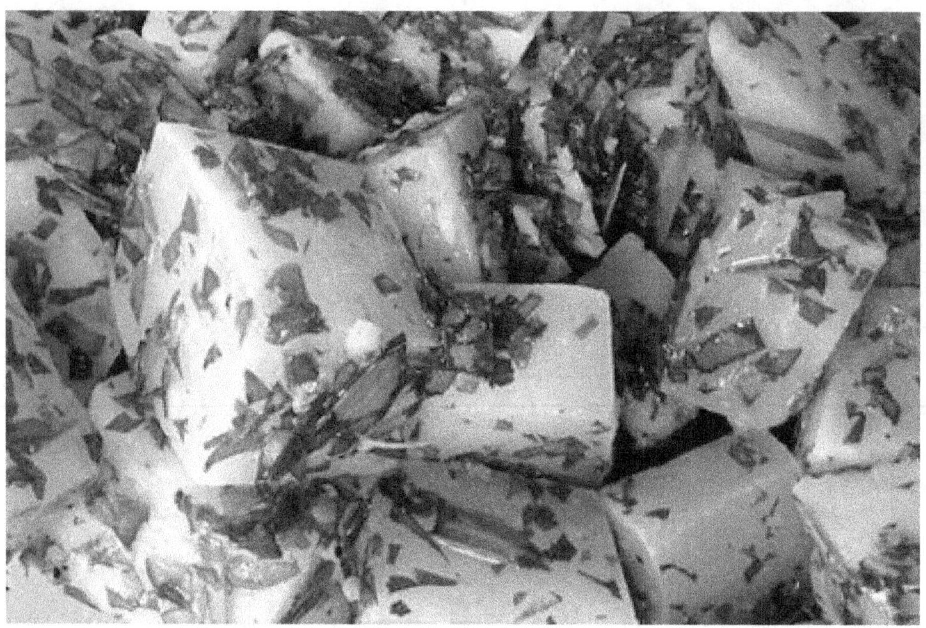

Ingredients for 4 portions

- 100 g   Goat cheese, hard cheese
- 2 stems Tarragon, possibly a little more, depending on the size
- 5 stems Parsley, smooth
- 1 Garlic cloves
- 2 tbsp. olive oil
- 1 splash   lemon juice
- salt
- Pepper, black, freshly ground

Preparation

Total time approx. 3 hours 20 minutes

Dice the cheese, pluck the leaves from the tarragon, finely chop the parsley, and mash the clove of garlic, olive oil and lemon juice. Season with a little salt (caution, not too much) and pepper, pour over the cheese and mix well.

Let the whole thing steep for a few hours. Before serving, remove from the refrigerator so that the cheese reaches room temperature.

You can also use sheep cheese,

DANISH ROAST FILLET WITH MUSTARD SAUCE

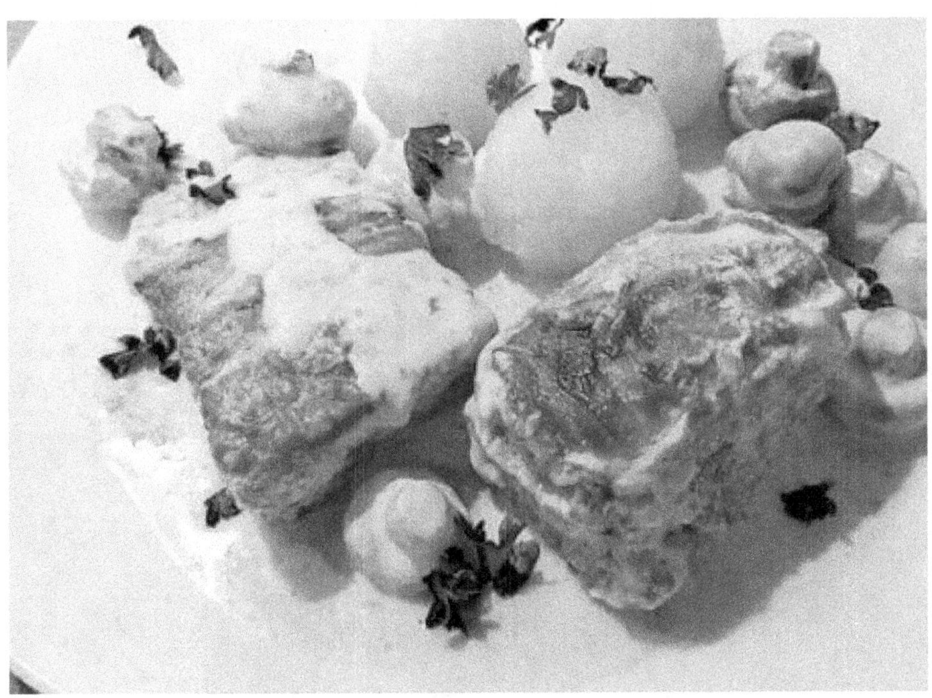

Ingredients for 4 portions

- 750 g   Pork
- 2 tbsp. Flour
- 1 teaspoon   salt
- ½ tsp   Pepper, white
- 250 g   Mushrooms, fresh
- 40 g   butter
- 2 Tea spoons   Mustard, lighter
- 1 cup   water
- 100 g   double cream
- 1 tbsp. tarragon

Preparation

Total time approx. 35 minutes

1. Remove tendons and fat from the fillets. Cut four thick slices out of it and flatten them slightly. Mix the flour, salt and pepper and turn the pieces of meat inside. Tap well so that no breading gets into the fat.
2. Brown the butter, fry the pieces of meat on high heat for 2 minutes on each side, switch back to medium heat. Continue frying for 1 - 2 minutes per side and keep warm.
3. Briefly steam the mushrooms in a saucepan in hot butter. Add the mustard to the meat butter and stir well. Stir in the water, the liquid of the mushrooms and the double cream cheese until the cheese has melted. Season the sauce spicy with salt and pepper and add the mushrooms.

4. Place half of the sauce on a preheated plate, place the pieces of meat on top and pour the rest of the sauce over the meat.

KASSEL

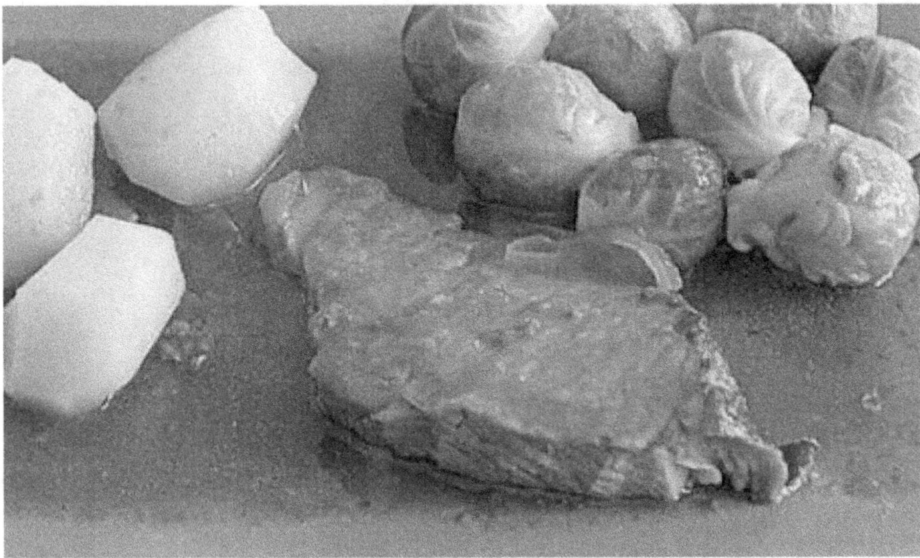

Ingredients for 4 portions

- 1 kg   Kessler (comb or neck)
- 4 large ones   Onion
- 2 tbsp. Margarine or clarified butter
- 1½ liters   water
- Salt and pepper
- Sauce binders, darker

Preparation

Total time approx. 20 minutes

1. First cut the onions into large cubes. Melt the margarine or clarified butter in a large saucepan and fry the Kessler vigorously on all sides. Then take the smoked pork out of the pot and set aside on a plate.
2. Now put the onions in the pot and let them brown. When the onions are lightly browned, put the smoked pork back into the pot and pour in the water - about enough to cover 2/3 of the meat. Bring to the boil and simmer for about 60 minutes over medium heat in a closed saucepan.
3. Season to taste and salt if necessary, as the salinity of the cashier is always different. After the braising season, season again and season with salt and pepper.
4. Take out the smoked pork and cut into slices. Thicken the liquid with the sauce binder and put the sliced slices back into the sauce. You also need boiled potatoes or pasta.

TUSCAN FILLET POT

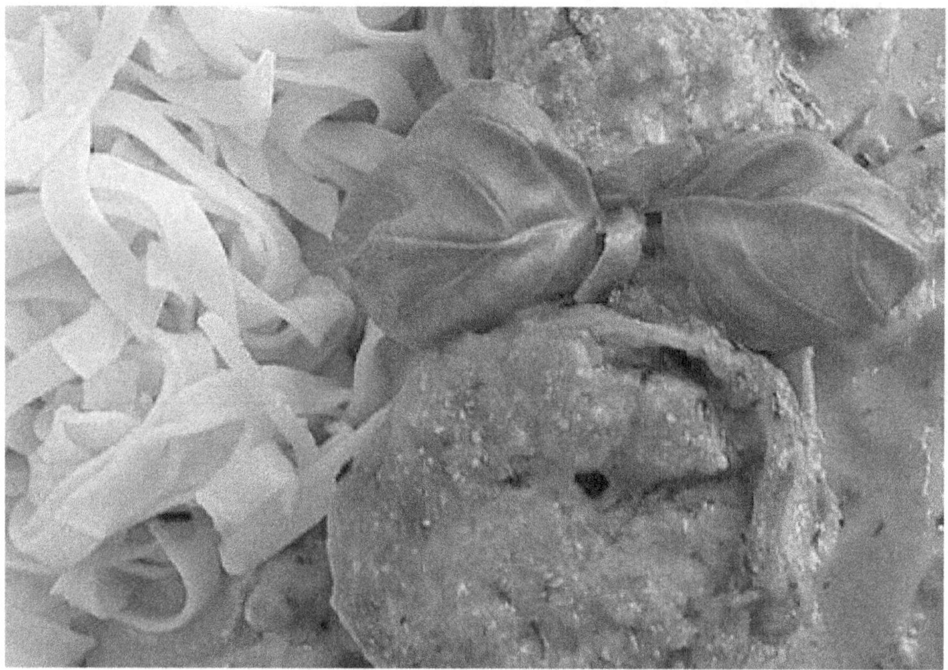

Ingredients for 4 portions

- 500 g   Pork
- 1 pack   Bacon
- 2 cups   whipped cream
- 1 can   tomato paste
- 300 g   Tomatoes
- Tomato ketchup
- 2 toes   garlic
- Paprika
- Cayenne pepper
- Chili powder
- Salt and pepper
- Rosemary
- Thyme
- Basil
- Butter
- Bread crumbs

Preparation

Total time approx. 40 minutes

1. Wash the meat and pat dry and divide into medallions.
2. Grease a baking dish and place the pieces of fillet wrapped with the bacon close together.
3. Preheat the oven to 180-200 ° C.

4. Now heat the cream in a saucepan. Quarter the tomatoes and stir into the cream with the tomato paste and some ketchup. Squeeze the garlic and add to the cream mixture. Season the whole thing with the spices and herbs.
5. Now bring to the boil briefly and pour hot over the fillet pieces. Put a few flakes of butter on top and sprinkle with a few breadcrumbs.
6. Bake in the oven for about 40 minutes at 200 ° C.
7. Fresh baguette tastes best with it.

INSALATA CAPRESE

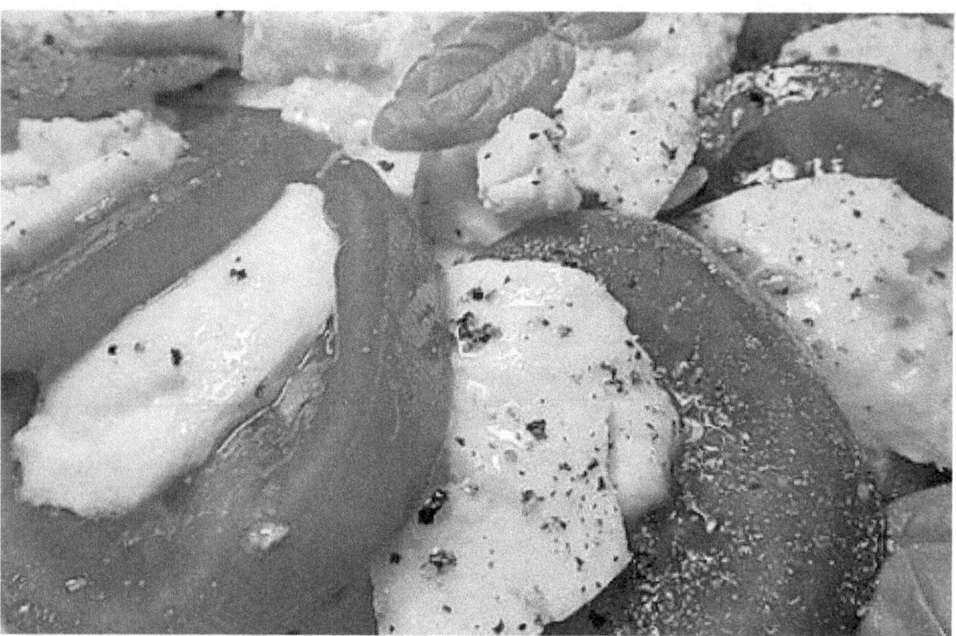

Ingredients for 2 portions

- 1 ball   Mozzarella, (buffalo mozzarella)
- 1 Meat tomato
- 1 bunchbasil
- Salt and pepper
- Olive oil, virgin, extra virgin (cold pressed)

Preparation

1   Total time approx. 10 minutes
2   Cut the buffalo mozzarella into thin slices. Wash, clean and slice the tomato. Clean the basil, pluck the leaves and cut into thin strips (chiffonade).
3   Arrange the tomatoes and mozzarella on a plate, season with salt and pepper. Drizzle with cold-pressed olive oil and garnish with the basil. Serve immediately.

SPICY TYROLEAN VEAL SLICED

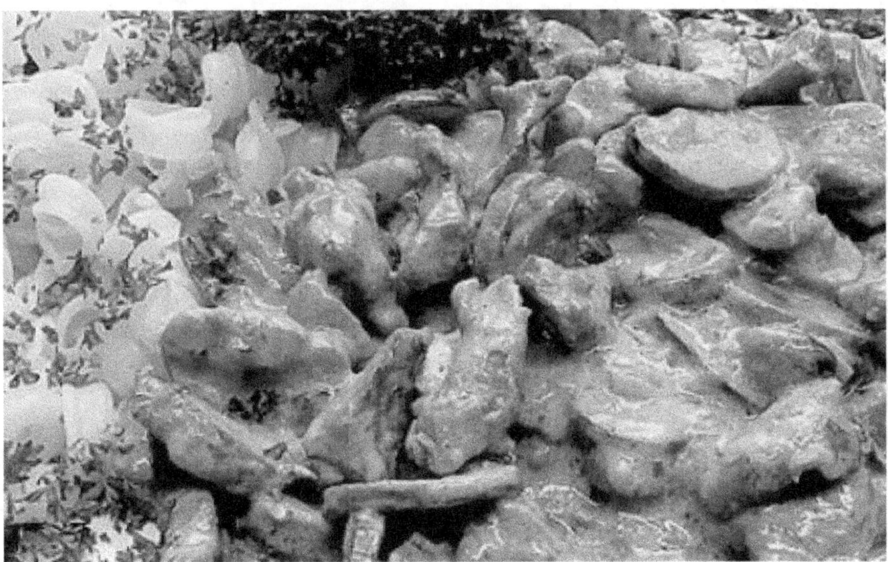

Ingredients for 4 portions

- ¾ kg   veal cutlet
- 1 Onion
- 250 g   mushrooms
- 70 g   bacon
- Oil
- 250 ml Whipped cream
- 125 g   Crème fraiche Cheese
- 100 g   Gorgonzola
- 1 tbsp. mustard
- 3 cl   Cognac or brandy
- Paprika
- Salt and pepper
- Curry powder
- Parsley, chopped

Preparation

Total time approx. 30 minutes

Cut the meat into strips. Peel the onion and cut it into small cubes together with the bacon. Clean the mushrooms and cut them into leaves.

Fry the meat quickly in hot oil, then remove. Then sweat the onion and bacon in the pan. Add the mushrooms and fry briefly. Deglaze with brandy and pour in whipped cream. Bring to the boil, then stir in the crème fraiche. Cut the gorgonzola into small pieces, add and melt in the sauce. Season with salt, pepper, mustard and a little curry powder (not too much). Finally add the meat again, warm briefly in the sauce and refine with parsley.

MOUSE HERB (LAYER HERB)

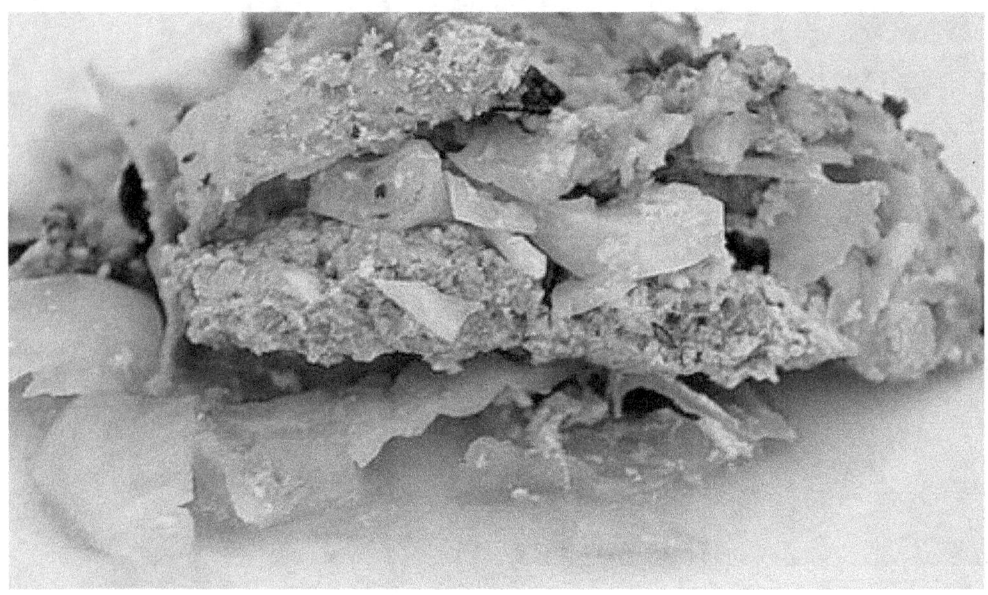

Ingredients for 8 portions

- 1 kg   minced meat
- 2 Onion
- 400 ml broth
- 1 head white cabbage
- Caraway seeds, whole or ground
- Salt and pepper
- Possibly.   Gravy
- Possibly.   Sour cream

Preparation

Total time approx. 30 minutes

1   Season the mince with salt and pepper. Add the onion and cumin. Quarter the cabbage, cut out the stalk and cut it into fine strips.

2   Cover the bottom of a large saucepan with a layer of cabbage. Then add a layer of hack, another layer of cabbage, etc. Repeat the whole thing until everything is used up. The last, top layer must be herb.

3   Pour the broth over it. Simmer everything on medium heat for 45 min. At the end, pour off some of the broth and tie it with gravy (or sour cream). Boiled potatoes are suitable as a side dish.

ITALIAN BOLOGNESE SAUCE

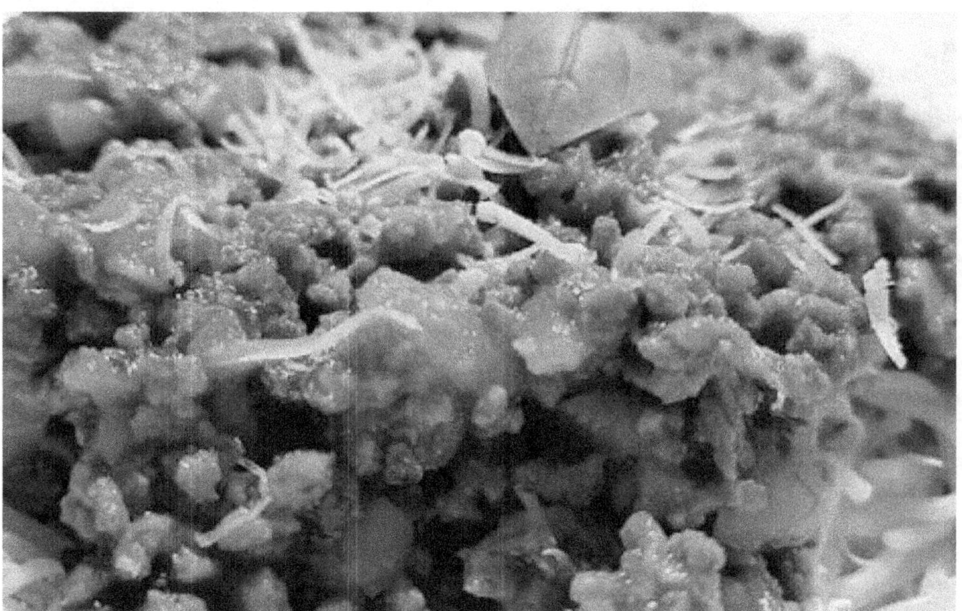

Ingredients for 4 portions

- 300 g   Beef, roughly chopped
- 150 g   Pork belly, finely chopped
- 50 g   Carrot, finely diced
- 50 g   Celery, finely diced
- 50 g   Onion, finely diced
- 300 g   Tomato, mashed or peeled, canned
- ½ glass Red wine, approx. 100 ml
- 1 glass Whole milk, approx. 200 ml
- Possibly.   Cream, approx. 100 ml
- Beef broth, liquid
- Olive oil or butter
- Salt and pepper

Preparation

Total time approx. 2 hours 45 minutes

1   Let the bacon cut into cubes and then finely chopped in a thick-walled pot with a diameter of about 20 cm. Then gently fry 3 tablespoons of oil or 50 g of butter and the finely diced vegetables. Add the beef and mix well with a ladle until well browned. Mix in the wine gently until the liquid has completely evaporated. Add the tomatoes, put the lid on the pan and let the sauce cook slowly for about 2 hours.

2   Add the broth if necessary. Add the milk towards the end to reduce the acidity of the tomatoes. Season with salt and pepper. When the sauce is ready, you can add cream, depending on your taste.

HAM - CHEESE - CREAM - SAUCE

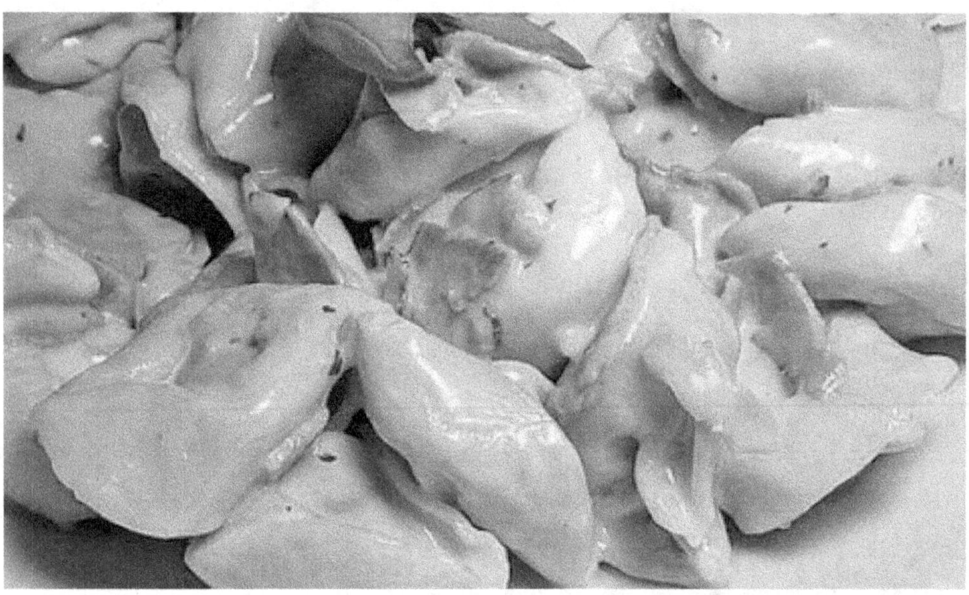

Ingredients for 4 portions

- 200 g   Cooked ham, finely diced
- 100 g   Processed cheese, (herbal processed cheese)
- 200 g   cream
- 20 g   butter
- salt and pepper

Preparation

Total time approx. 15 minutes

Melt the butter in a saucepan over medium heat and stir the ham in it for 2 minutes. Then deglaze with the cream and melt the processed cheese in it. Bring the sauce to a boil and season with salt and pepper.

Tastes great with all types of pasta or simply with potatoes or vegetables.

SHRIMP SKEWERS

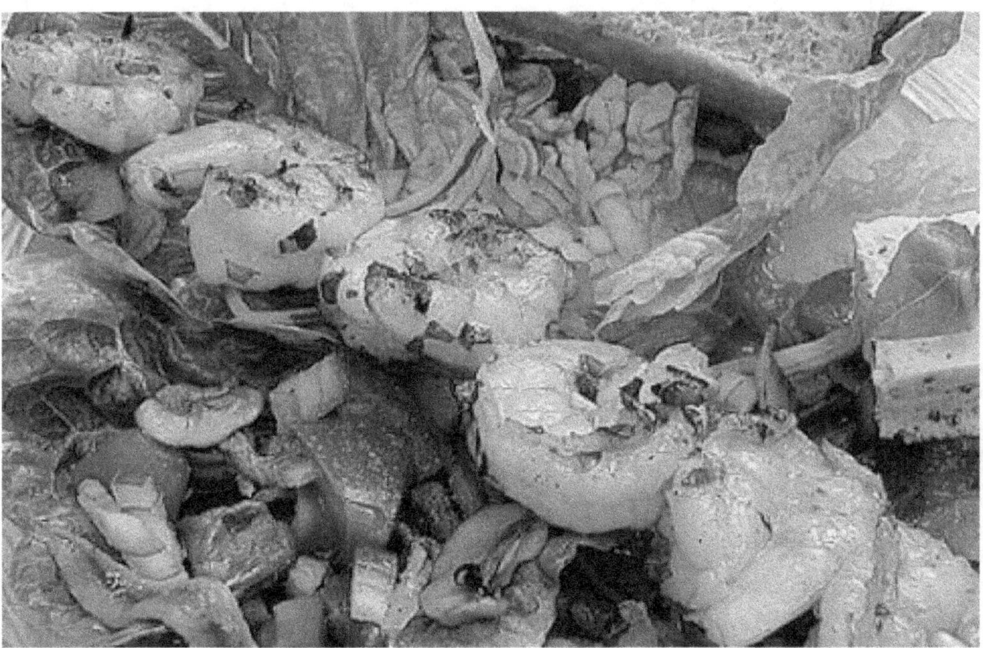

Ingredients for 3 portions

- 250 g   Shrimp (approx. 18)
- ½ bundle   basil
- Garlic cloves)
- 2 tbsp. olive oil
- Salt and pepper

Preparation

Total time approx. 20 minutes

- Wash and chop the basil. Peel the clove of garlic, press through and mix with basil, olive oil, salt and pepper. Mix the prawns with the marinade and let them steep. Then put on three skewers and brush with the rest of the marinade. Grill under turns or fry in a grill pan.
- In addition: Bread and herb butter
- The shrimp not only taste as a starter, but also when barbecuing or on a salad you have made yourself! Great in summer!

SWISS STYLE PORK FILLETS

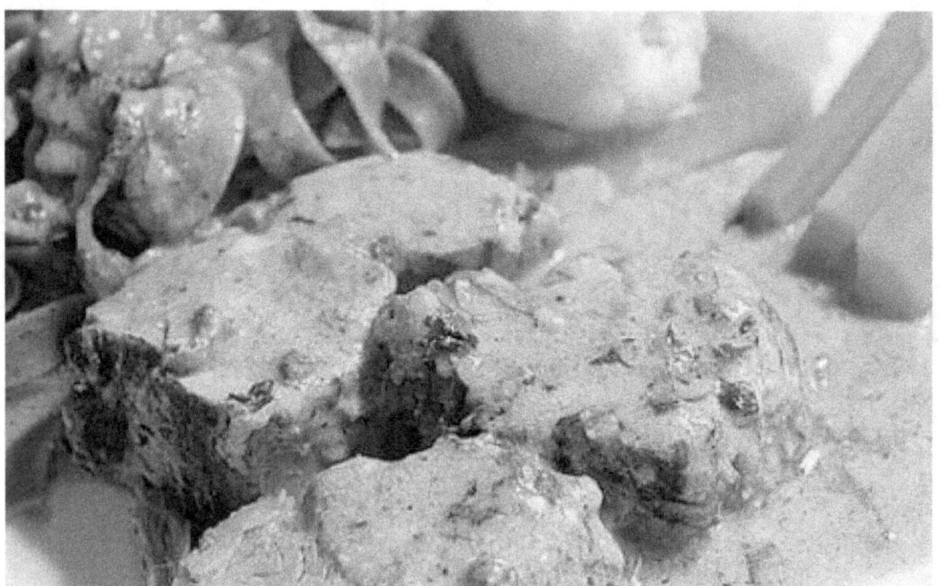

Ingredients for 4 portions

- 200 g   Cheese, in thick slices
- Pork fillet, each about 400 g
- 1 teaspoon   Pepper, black from the mill
- 2 Tea spoons   Paprika powder, hot
- 1 teaspoon   Dried thyme
- 1 teaspoon   Oregano, dried
- Salt
- 2 tbsp. clarified butter
- 125 ml Meat soup
- 200 g   Crème fraiche Cheese
- 1 bunchParsley, smooth
- Lemon juice

Preparation

Total time approx. 20 minutes

1   Debark the cheese and cut into about 2 cm long sticks. Cut slits all around in the fillets and press in the cheese sticks.
2   Mix the pepper with the paprika, thyme, oregano and very little salt and turn the peppered pork fillets into it.
3   Heat the clarified butter in a roaster and fry the pork fillets all around. Deglaze with the meat broth, stir in the crème fraiche and cover and simmer for about 25 minutes.
4   Wash the parsley, shake dry, pluck and chop finely. Season the sauce with salt, pepper and lemon juice and finally stir in the parsley.
5   Serve the fillets sliced.

6   Narrow ribbon pasta or mashed potatoes with fresh herbs and lettuce are suitable as a side dish.

TIP: The type of cheese can be exchanged as you like, and various cheese residues are also very suitable for this.

GREEK PASTORAL CREAM

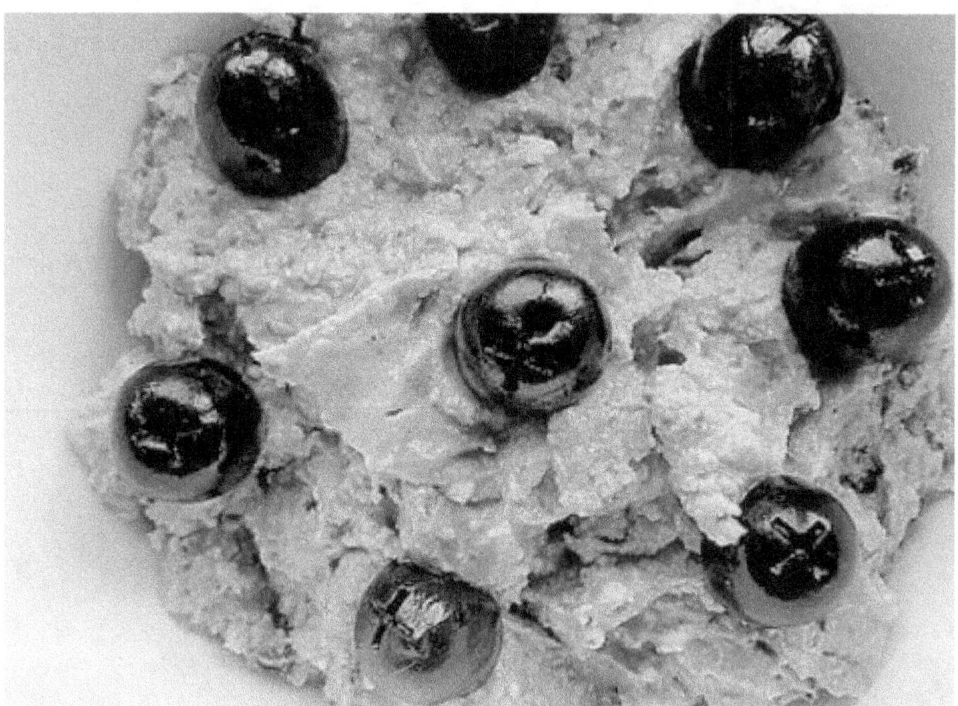

Ingredients for 8 portions

- 20 Olives, black
- 4 toes garlic
- 400 g feta cheese
- 200 g Butter, soft
- 5 tbsp. milk
- 4 tbsp. tomato paste
- Salt
- Black pepper
- Oregano

Preparation

Total time approx. 10 minutes

1 Core the olives and slice them, press the garlic through them. Finely chop the cheese with a fork and mix with the soft butter, then gradually add milk, tomato paste, spices to taste and finally add the olives and garlic. Let it steep a little before serving.
2 Tastes great on baguette, farmhouse bread or as a dip for raw food.

PICKLED ZUCCHINI ROLLS

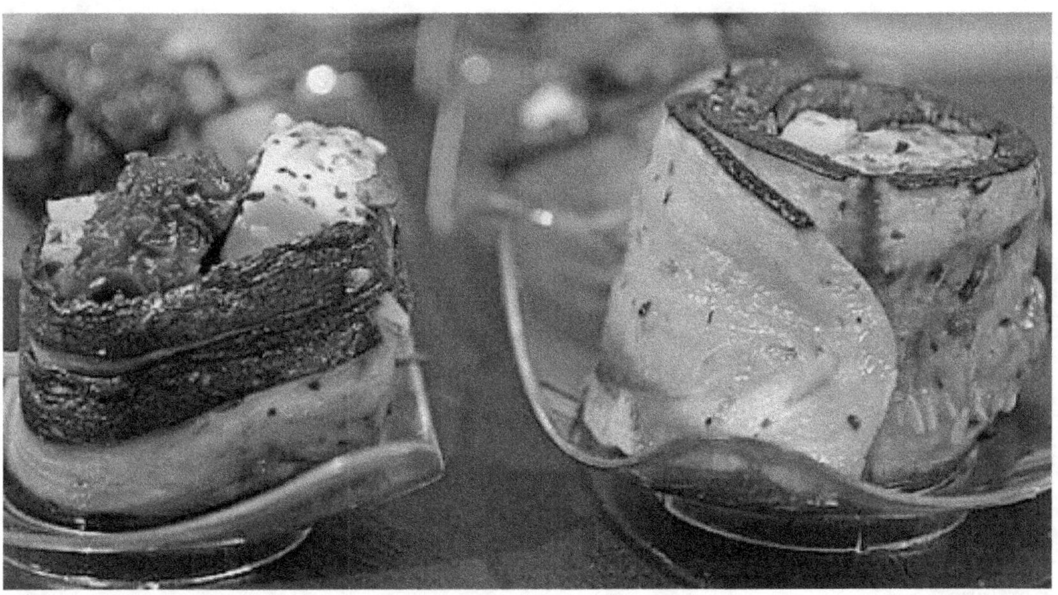

Ingredients for 4 portions

- Zucchini, thinly sliced
- 200 g   Feta cheese
- 3 Garlic cloves
- 1 cup   olive oil
- 2 Tea spoons   Herbs, Italian, of your choice
- 2 Chili
- 2 tbsp. balsamic

Preparation

Total time approx. 35 minutes

1   Wash, dry and cut the zucchini lengthways into thin slices. Then fry in portions in heated olive oil.
2   Dice the feta cheese. Fill the fried zucchini slices with it and roll up. Put in a slightly higher form. Chop the cloves of garlic and chili pepper and spread them on the rolls. Sprinkle herbs over it and drizzle the balsamic vinegar over it.
3   Now put the mold in the fridge for 3 days until it is served.

GAMBAS WITH GARLIC

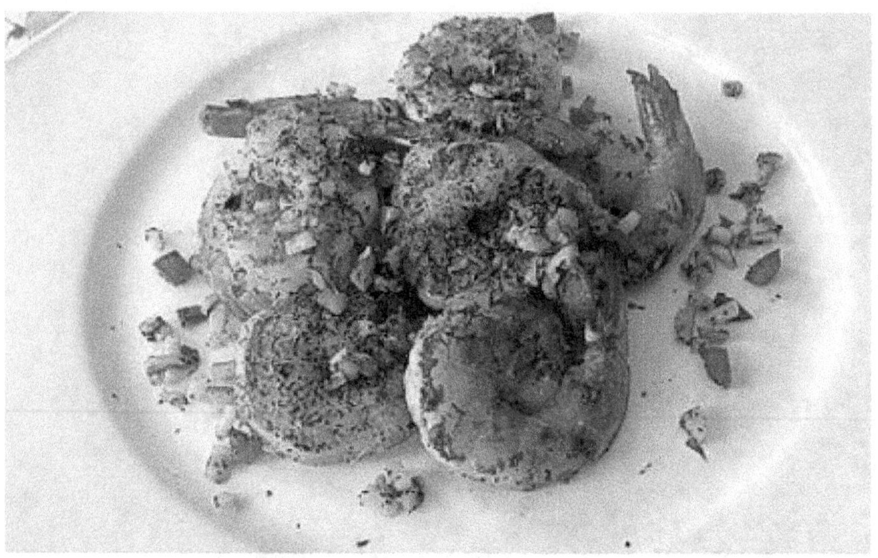

Ingredients for 4 portions

- 500 g   Gambas, ready to cook
- 1 Chili pepper, red
- 5 Garlic cloves
- Olive oil
- Salt and pepper
- 1 bunchParsley, finely chopped

Preparation

Total time approx. 30 minutes

1. Core the chili and cut into strips. Heat the olive oil in a coated or cast iron pan. Add the garlic, chili and the prawns and sear for 2 minutes. Season and sprinkle the parsley on top before serving.

    A glass of sherry goes with it!

VIENNESE ROAST WITH MUSHROOMS

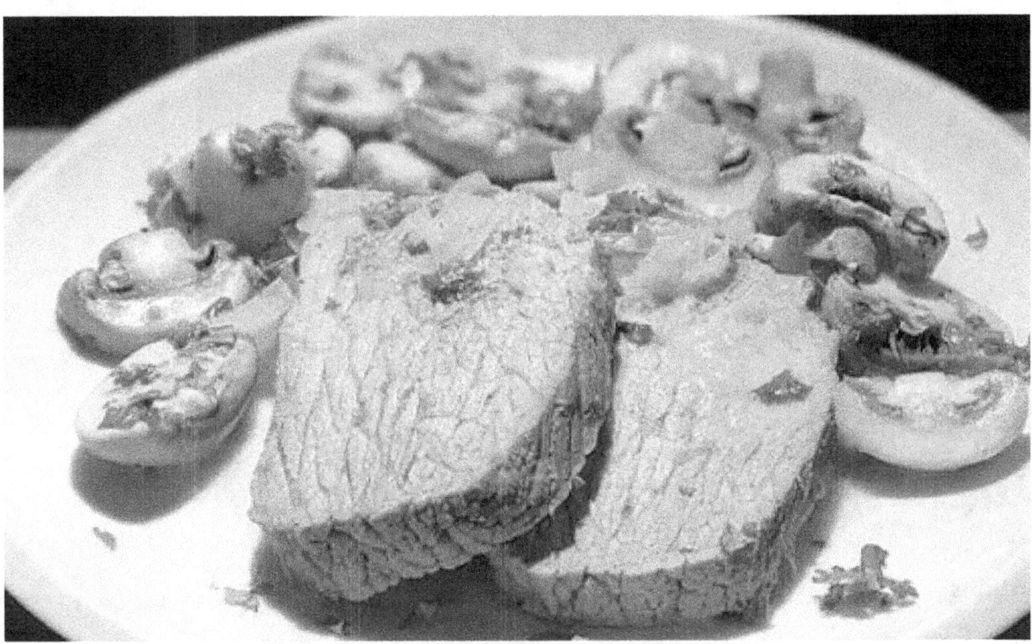

Ingredients for 4 portions

- 1 kg   Roast veal (nut)
- 60 g   clarified butter
- Shallot
- ¼ liter   White wine, dry (Riesling)
- 250 g   sour cream
- 80 g   bacon
- 400 g   Mushrooms, e.g. chanterelles or mushrooms
- Salt and pepper
- Parsley, freshly chopped

Preparation

Total time approx. 1 hour 30 minutes

2   Rub the meat with salt and pepper. Heat 40 g clarified butter in a casserole and sear the meat all over. Add the shallots and fry briefly. Pour in the Riesling, cover and stew everything for about 50 minutes.

3   Remove the meat and keep it warm. Stir the sour cream into the roast stock and season the sauce with salt.

4   Fry the diced bacon in a pan in 20 g clarified butter. Add the cleaned mushrooms and season with salt and pepper. Steam in the pan for 15 minutes.

5   Carve the roast veal in slices and arrange on a plate. Sprinkle with the sauce, add the mushrooms all around on the plate and sprinkle with freshly chopped parsley.

6   Serve with serviette dumplings or roasted potatoes.

CHICKEN SKEWERS

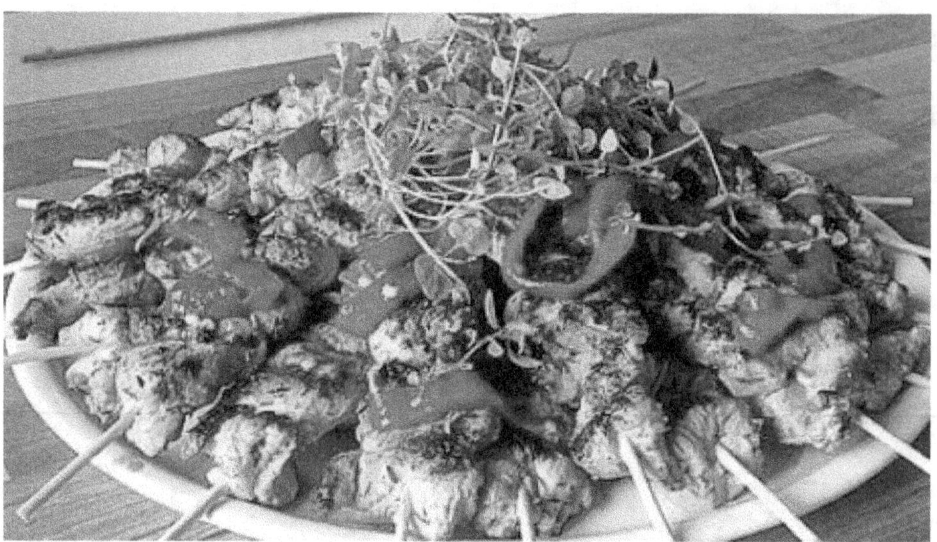

Ingredients for 4 portions

- 500 g   chicken breasts

For the marinade:

- Lemon, juice from it
- 4 toes   garlic
- 1 tbsp. Paprika powder, noble sweet
- 1 tbsp. thyme
- 1 pinch cumin
- 2 Tea spoons   salt

Preparation

Total time approx. 8 hours 30 minutes

- Cut the chicken into small pieces. Crush the garlic and sprinkle with salt. Add all other ingredients and arrange for a marinade. Leave the chicken pieces in it overnight (in the refrigerator).
- Put pieces of meat on the skewers and keep a little marinade between each piece. Then sear well and serve hot or cold.

ITALIAN LAMB RAGOUT

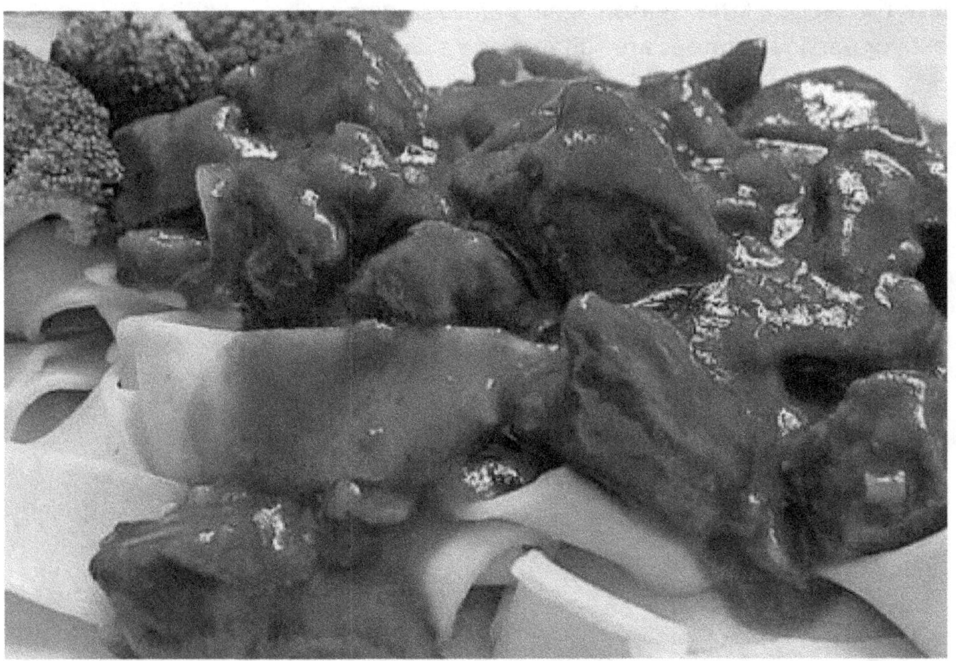

Ingredients for 4 portions

- 600 g   Boneless lamb (leg or shoulder)
- 80 g   Bacon, streaky
- 1 Onion
- 2 Garlic cloves
- Olive oil
- Clarified butter
- 1½ tbsp.   Flour
- 200 ml Meat soup
- 200 ml Red wine, drier
- 2 tbsp. tomato paste
- 1 pinch cinnamon
- Salt and pepper from the mill

Preparation

Total time approx. 20 minutes

1   Cut the lamb into cubes. Finely dice onions and garlic. Cut the bacon into small strips.
2   Sauté the onions and bacon in a mixture of oil and clarified butter in a roasting pan, add the garlic and fry briefly, then take everything out of the roasting pan. Add the lamb and sear on all sides. Add the onion mixture again, dust everything with the flour, sweat briefly and then deglaze with broth. Season with salt and pepper, cover and braise on a low flame. Stir occasionally.

3   After 30 minutes pour in the red wine, stir in the tomato paste and season with a pinch of cinnamon. Braise for another 30 minutes. Shortly before the end of the cooking time, remove the lid and reduce the sauce a little. Season again before serving.

4   Wide ribbon pasta or parsley potatoes are suitable as a side dish.

SHRIMP WITH GARLIC, OIL AND CHILLI SAUCE

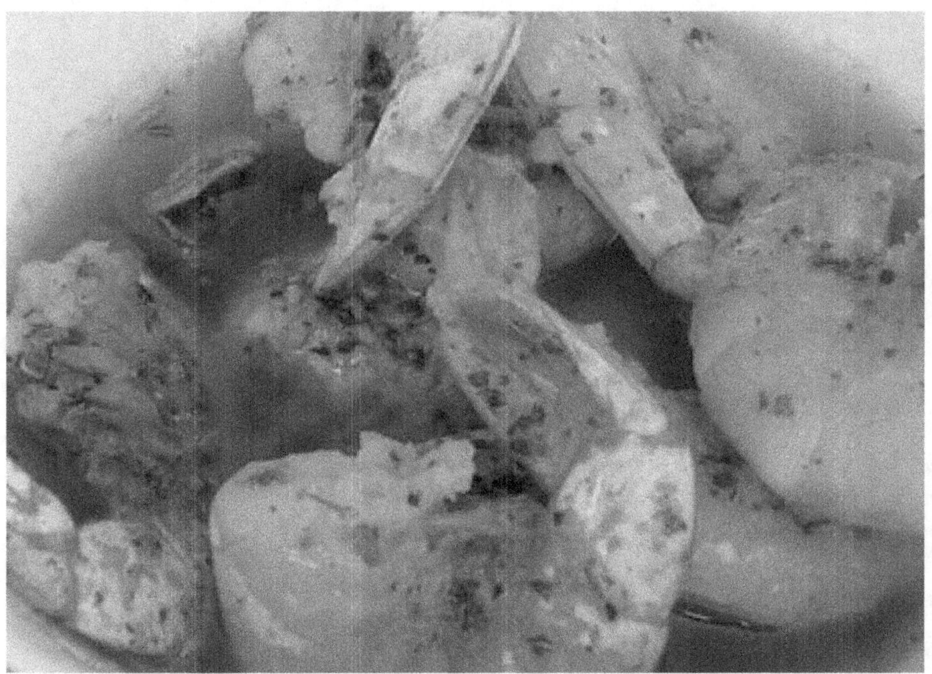

Ingredients for 4 portions

- 6 tbsp. olive oil
- 4 Clove of garlic, crushed
- 2 pepper, dried red, seeded and crumbled
- 500 g   King prawns, unpeeled raw
- Sea-salt

Preparation

Total time approx. 15 minutes

1   Heat the oil in a pan. Add garlic and chilies and cook for 1 to 2 minutes. Then add the shrimp and sea salt to taste. Fry the shrimp vigorously for 2 minutes, turning constantly.
2   Serve the prawns on preheated serving plates, along with good bread to take the sauce.

FILLED MEATBALLS GREEK STYLE

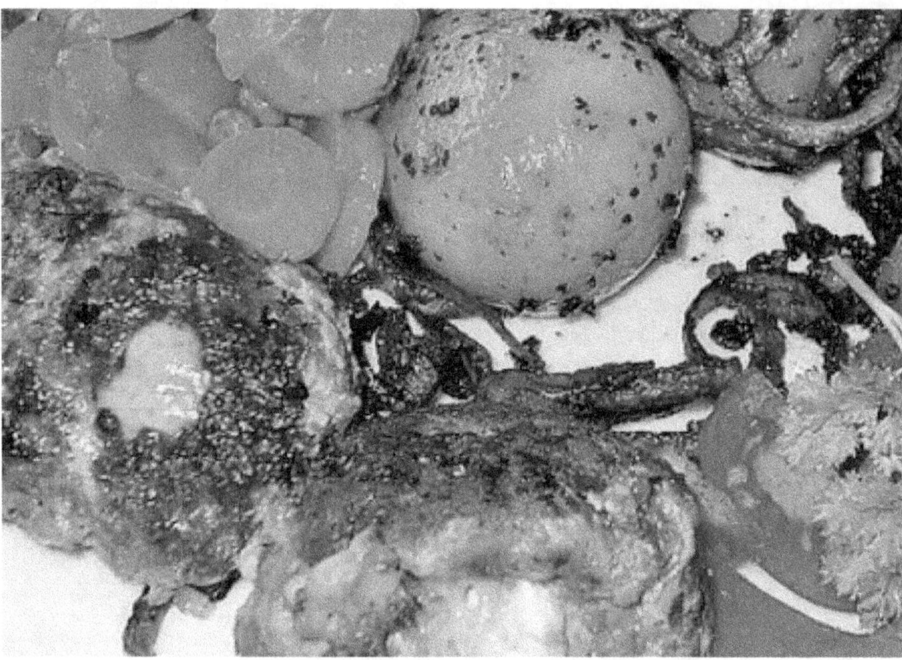

Ingredients for 3 portions

- 500 g   Minced meat, mixed
- 1 small Onion
- 1 teaspoon   Salt, to taste
- Pepper, black from the mill
- 1 teaspoon   Marjoram, fresh or dried
- 1 teaspoon   Oregano, fresh or dried
- Rosemary, fresh or dried
- Egg
- 3 tbsp. breadcrumbs
- Garlic cloves
- 100 g   Sheep cheese or
- Feta cheese
- 1 teaspoon   Paprika powder, noble sweet
- 3 tbsp. Oil or fat for frying

Preparation

Total time approx. 15 minutes

1   Finely chop the onion and garlic. Now put the minced meat, the eggs, the spices, garlic, onions and the breadcrumbs in a bowl and mix well. Let the meat mass soak in the refrigerator for 20 minutes.

2   Take the mass out of the fridge again. Take 2 tablespoons of meat mass in your hand and form a pound. Press a depression in the middle of the Klopses and place a small piece of sheep's

cheese in it. Squeeze the sides of the beater together and form an oval elongated meatball. Do the same with the rest of the meat until the ingredients are used up.

3   Now fry the meatballs in a pan with hot oil for 20 minutes on both sides over medium heat. My rosemary baked potatoes and my delicious farmer's salad go very well with this.

FISH AND CHIPS

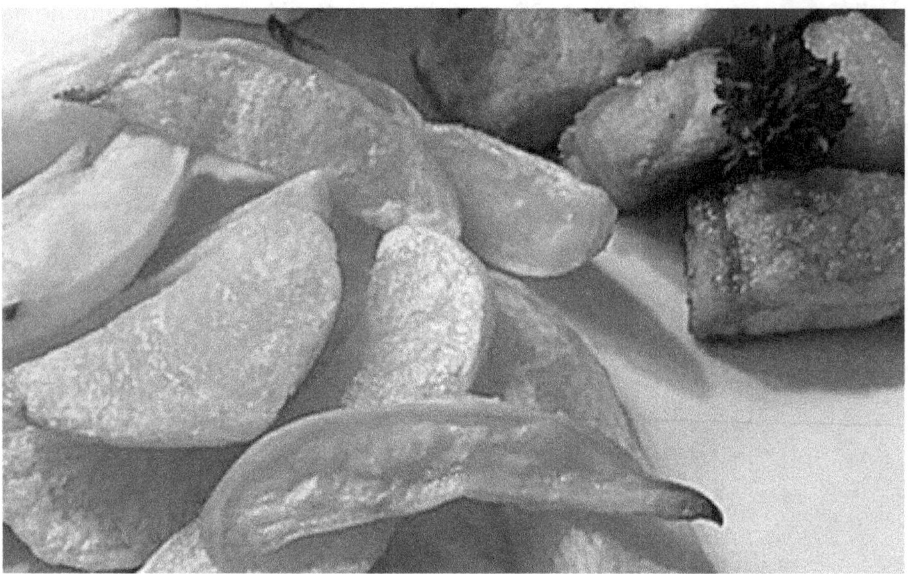

Ingredients for 4 portions

- 165 g   Flour, self-propelled, (Self Raising Flour)
- ½ tsp   salt
- ½ tsp   baking powder
- ½ tsp   turmeric
- 200 ml wheat beer
- 1.3 kg   Potato, large, mealy boiling
- 700 g   Cod fillet or haddock fillet, without skin
- 2 liters vegetable oil
- 2 Lemons
- Sea-salt
- Pepper, freshly ground
- Vinegar, English

Preparation

Total time approx. 1 hour 45 minutes

1   Sift 125 g of self-propelling flour with the salt, baking powder and turmeric (turmeric) into a bowl. Then you press a hole in the middle and gradually stir in half of the beer with a whisk, so that a firm dough is formed. Then you stir in the other half of the beer. You cover the bowl and let the dough steep in the fridge for 1 hour.

2   In the meantime, peel the potatoes and cut them into thick strips about 1.5 cm in diameter in order to obtain thick chips. The chips are pre-fried either in the deep fryer or in a deep pan with sufficient oil at 190 ° C. When they are just done, but not yet crispy, you take them out and let them cool.

3   Pat the fish dry and cut into 4 large pieces. Season with sea salt and pepper from all sides. Store in the refrigerator until preparation.

4   Deep-fry the pre-fried chips at 190 ° C until they are crispy on the outside. Keep warm in the oven at 50 - 60 ° C.

5   Get the fish and dough out of the fridge. Dust the fish thoroughly with the remaining flour. Then dip the fish in the dough so that it is completely covered and then carefully place it in the oil, which is approx. 150 ° C to 160 ° C. Deep-fry for about 4 minutes until golden brown and crispy. Dab with kitchen paper and serve with the chips and lemon wedges and the vinegar.

ROAST CRUST IN HONEY - THYME SAUCE

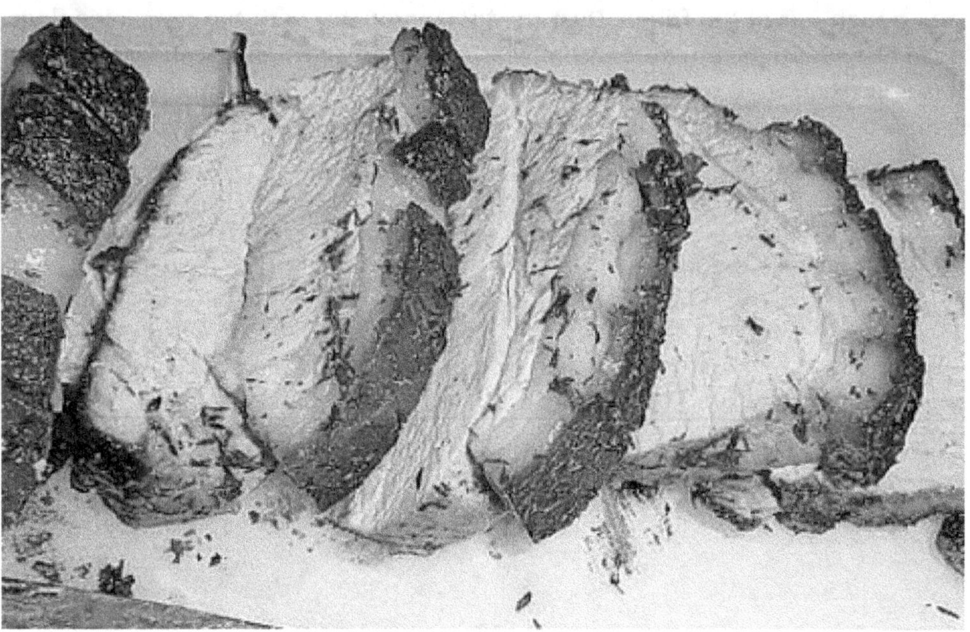

Ingredients for 4 portions

- 1 kg   Pork (pork shoulder with rind), sprayed
- 2 Tea spoons   mustard
- Thyme
- 1 toe   garlic
- 250 g   butter
- 4 tbsp. honey
- Pepper

Preparation

Total time approx. 1 hour

1   Bring the butter to room temperature, place in a mixing bowl and preheat the oven to 200 °
C. Carve the rind crosswise with a sharp knife (approx. 2 mm deep), salt and pepper the meat
and sauté all around. Mix the butter with approx. 4 tablespoons honey, 2 teaspoons mustard,
sufficient thyme and the crushed clove of garlic. Season this marinade with salt and the other
ingredients. Brush the meat thickly with the marinade and put it in the oven in a closed
roaster. Make sure that there is always enough water in the roaster. Brush the marinade onto
the rind from time to time. After about 1 1/2 to 2 hours in the oven, place the roast on the
top rail and switch on the top heat. Remove the lid from the roaster.

Tip: You can also brush the crust with salt water at the end, which makes it nice and crunchy.